DRUGS
The Straight Facts

Weight-Loss Drugs

DRUGS The Straight Facts

■ DRUGS
The Straight Facts

Weight-Loss Drugs

Suellen May

Consulting Editor
David J. Triggle, Ph.D.
University Professor
School of Pharmacy and Pharmaceutical Sciences
State University of New York at Buffalo

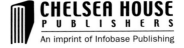
CHELSEA HOUSE
P U B L I S H E R S
An imprint of Infobase Publishing

Drugs The Straight Facts: Weight-Loss Drugs

Chelsea House
An imprint of Infobase Publishing
132 West 31st Street
New York NY 10001

Library of Congress Cataloging-in-Publication Data
May, Suellen.
  Weight loss drugs / Suellen May, David J. Triggle.
    p. cm. — (Drugs, the straight facts)
  Includes bibliographical references and index.
  ISBN-13: 978-1-60413-204-5 (alk. paper)
  ISBN-10: 1-60413-204-3 (alk. paper)
  1. Appetite depressants. 2. Weight loss preparations. 3. Weight loss. I. Triggle, D. J. II. Title. III. Series.
  RM332.3.M39 2009
  615'.78—dc22

                          2008040953

Table of Contents

The Use and Abuse of Drugs

For thousands of years, humans have used a variety of sources with which to cure their ills, cast out devils, promote their well-being, relieve their misery, and control their fertility. Until the beginning of the twentieth century, the agents used were all of natural origin, including many derived from plants as well as elements such as antimony, sulfur, mercury, and arsenic. The sixteenth-century alchemist and physician Paracelsus used mercury and arsenic in his treatment of syphilis, worms, and other diseases that were common at that time; his cure rates, however, remain unknown. Many drugs used today have their origins in natural products. Antimony derivatives, for example, are used in the treatment of the nasty tropical disease leish-maniasis. These plant-derived products represent molecules that have been "forged in the crucible of evolution" and con-tinue to supply the scientist with molecular scaffolds for new drug development.

Our story of modern drug discovery may be considered to start with the German physician and scientist Paul Ehrlich, often called the father of chemotherapy. Born in 1854, Ehrlich became interested in the ways in which synthetic dyes, then becoming a major product of the German fine chemical industry, could stain selectively certain tissues and components of cells. He reasoned that such dyes might form the basis for drugs that could interact selectively with diseased or foreign cells and organisms. One of Ehrlich's early successes was his development of the arsenical "606"—patented under the name Salvarsan—as a treatment for syphilis. Ehrlich's goal was to create a "magic bullet," a drug that would target only the diseased cell or the invading dis-ease-causing organism and have no effect on healthy cells and tissues. In this he was not successful, but his great research did lay the groundwork for the successes of the twentieth century, including the discovery of the sulfonamides and the antibiotic penicillin. The latter agent saved countless lives during World War II. Ehrlich, like many scientists, was an optimist. On the eve of World War I, he wrote, "Now that the liability to, and danger of, disease are to a large extent circumscribed—the efforts of chemotherapeutics are directed as far as possible to fill up the gaps left in this ring." As we shall see in this volume, it is neither the first nor the last time that science has proclaimed its victory over Nature only to have to see this optimism dashed in the light of some freshly emerging infection.

From these advances, however, has come the vast array of drugs that are available to the modern physician. We are increasingly close to Ehrlich's magic bullet: Drugs can now target very specific molecular defects in a number of cancers, and doctors today have the ability to investigate the human genome to more effectively match the drug and the patient. In the next one to two decades, it is almost certain that the cost of "reading" an individual genome will be sufficiently cheap that, at least in the developed world, such personalized medicines will become the norm. The development of such drugs, however, is extremely costly and raises significant social issues, including equity in the delivery of medical treatment.

The twenty-first century will continue to produce major advances in medicines and medicine delivery. Nature is, however, a resilient foe. Diseases and organisms develop resistance to existing drugs, and new drugs must constantly be developed. (This is particularly true for anti-infective and anticancer agents.) Additionally, new and more lethal forms of existing infectious diseases can develop rapidly. With the ease of global travel, these illnesses can spread from Timbuktu to Toledo in fewer than 24 hours and become pandemics. Hence the current concerns about avian flu. Also, diseases that have previously been dormant or geographically circumscribed may suddenly break out worldwide. (Imagine, for example, a worldwide pandemic of Ebola disease, and how this event would totally overwhelm public health agencies.) Finally, there are serious concerns regarding the possibility of man-made epidemics occurring through the deliberate or accidental spread of disease agents—including manufactured agents, such as smallpox with enhanced lethality. It is therefore imperative that the search for new medicines continues.

All of us at some time in our life will take a medicine, even if it is only aspirin for a headache. For some individuals, drug use will be constant throughout life. As we age, we will likely be exposed to a variety of medications—from childhood vaccines to drugs to relieve pain caused by a terminal disease. It is not easy to get accurate and understandable information about the drugs that we consume to treat diseases and disorders. There are, of course, highly specialized volumes aimed at medical or scientific professionals. However, such texts require their readers to possess a sophisticated knowledge base and experience. Advertising on television is widely available but provides only fleeting information, usually about only a single drug and designed to market rather than inform. The intent of this series of books, Drugs: The Straight Facts, is to provide the lay reader with intelligent, readable, and accurate descriptions of drugs; an explanation of why and how they are used; and information about their limitations, their side effects, and their future. It is our hope that these books will provide readers with sufficient information to satisfy their immediate needs and to serve as an adequate base for further investigation and for asking intelligent questions of health care providers.

The present volume, *Weight-Loss Drugs,* discusses a group of drugs that are employed in the control of weight. The twenty-first century presents an ironic picture of a world population expanding simultaneously in both number and size. The ready availability of highly palatable, energy-dense foods has, together with major lifestyle changes, resulted in a population that is increasingly overweight or obese. This epidemic of weight increase is not confined to adults, but is also an increasingly serious problem with children. To be sure, this epidemic is not uniform—the world is still dramatically unequal, and the number of obese individuals is counterbalanced by an even greater number of people for whom the arrival of the next meal is uncertain.

How to tackle this global epidemic of obesity is a major problem. It is both a medical and a public health problem.

It is quite clear that public health measures must be a major component of any approach; and that these interventions, involving diet, exercise, and education, must start at an early age. Intervention with drugs will also be a part of an integrated approach, but the complexities of the physiological processes that control feeding behavior make this a very difficult task. The drugs that are available and that are discussed in this volume are far from satisfactory, and some have been associated with extremely serious side effects, including death, and virtually all are subject to abuse. Awareness of these limitations is a vital component of any effort to tackle the problems of overweight and obesity.

David J. Triggle, Ph.D.
University Professor
School of Pharmacy and Pharmaceutical Sciences
State University of New York at Buffalo

1
Weight, Obesity, and BMI

Obesity is a worldwide epidemic. Approximately one out of every three Americans is obese, according to the National Institutes of Health. Particularly disturbing is the increase of obesity in children. According to the Nemours Foundation, 10 percent of 2- to 5-year-olds and more than 15 percent of children between the ages of 6 and 19 are overweight.[1] In response to this trend and in consideration of the health risks of being overweight, **weight-loss drugs** are in great demand. Weight-loss drugs refer to any over-the-counter or prescription drug used for weight loss. Like any drug, these weight-loss aids present varying degrees of risk. Many doctors advise patients to assume the risks of these drugs even to experience the average 5- to 10-percent weight loss. This risk was grossly miscalculated, however, with drugs such as Redux and Fen-phen, which caused some consumers permanent heart and lung damage. This book will describe the health and emotional implications of being overweight, the biological mechanisms of weight-loss drugs, and the benefits and side effects of these drugs.

WEIGHT-LOSS DRUGS: PILLS AND SUPPLEMENTS

Weight-loss drugs are intended to enable patients to lose weight more effectively than diet or exercise alone by suppressing appetite, inhibiting the absorption of fat, or in some cases, increasing the metabolism slightly. Maximum weight loss as a direct result of the drugs will generally show results within the first six months. A patient could also lose weight due to the drugs after the first six months, but it will be a moderate weight loss. The length of time during which a person will continue to lose weight as a direct result of the weight-loss drug depends on how long it takes his or her body to adjust to the medication. Despite the efficacy of weight-loss drugs, the likelihood of losing significant weight without also increasing exercise or making dietary changes is unlikely. For this reason, patients should always incorporate at least some form of exercise and dieting as part of their weight-loss plan. Even if a patient's weight loss has leveled and he or she has reached a target weight, the individual must continue to take the medication to maintain the weight loss; this is controversial because some doctors believe the safety of taking many of these drugs for decades is not yet well known. We know that many weight-loss drugs cannot be taken long term, and therefore the patient must switch to another weight-loss drug, further increase exercise, or adjust his or her diet.

Weight-loss drugs are generally prescribed for people who are obese, not those who are slightly overweight or those looking to get ultra-slim. The most common guideline used to determine who is underweight, normal weight, overweight, or obese, is the body mass index (BMI). The body mass index is a guideline of how appropriate a person's weight is given his or her height. BMI is a number that represents weight divided by height squared. The Centers for Disease Control and Prevention (CDC) and the World Health Organization (WHO) define the weight status categories with BMI ranges for adults in the following table:

Table 1.1

BMI	Weight Status
Below 18.5	Underweight
18.5–24.9	Normal
25.0–29.9	Overweight
30.0–39.9	Obese

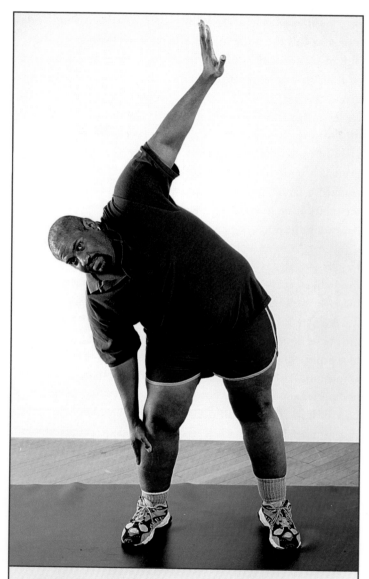

Figure 1.1 Weight-loss drugs may work by suppressing the appetite, inhibiting the body's absorption of fat, or boosting the body's metabolism slightly. These drugs are intended to support an overall weight-loss plan of making healthy diet choices and exercising. (© Custom Medical Stock Photo)

To illustrate what these numbers translate to in pounds, the following information demonstrates various BMI categories for a person who is 5'9" tall.

Table 1.2

Weight	BMI	Weight Status
124 lbs or less	Below 18.5	Underweight
125 lbs to 168 lbs	18.5 to 24.9	Normal
169 lbs to 202 lbs	25.0 to 29.9	Overweight
203 lbs or more	30 or higher	Obese[2]

There are two additional subcategories, morbidly obese and super morbidly obese. Morbidly obese represents people with a BMI of 40.0 to 49.9, and super morbidly obese refers to people with a BMI of 50.0 and above.

Assessing weight with BMI also has its critics in the medical community. The problem with BMI to determine a healthy weight is that is does not account for how much muscle a person has. An extremely muscular person may be considered overweight according to BMI but could be healthy and fit. Consider, for example, the basketball player Shaquille O'Neal. At 7'1" and 325 pounds, O'Neal's BMI is 31.6, which puts him in the "obese" category. Shaquille O'Neal is definitely not obese; he is extremely muscular, and therefore BMI is not a suitable evaluator of his health. A person also could have a normal BMI but be in poor nutritional health. Elderly people who have lost muscle due to inactivity might be considered a normal weight due to their BMI but in fact may have reduced nutritional reserves.

For children and teens (ages 2 through 19), the criterion for overweight is slightly different than for an adult. For children and teens, BMI age- and sex-specific percentiles are used because the amount of body fat changes with age, and

Body Mass Index (BMI)

Weight in pounds

Height	120	130	140	150	160	170	180	190	200	210	220	230	240	250
4'6"	29	31	34	36	39	41	43	46	48	51	53	56	58	60
4'8"	27	29	31	34	36	38	40	43	45	47	49	52	54	56
4'10"	25	27	29	31	34	36	38	40	42	44	46	48	50	52
5'0"	23	25	27	29	31	33	35	37	39	41	43	45	47	49
5'2"	22	24	26	27	29	31	33	35	37	38	40	42	44	46
5'4"	21	22	24	26	28	29	31	33	34	36	38	40	41	43
5'6"	19	21	23	24	26	27	29	31	32	34	36	37	39	40
5'8"	18	20	21	23	24	26	27	29	30	32	34	35	37	38
5'10"	17	19	20	22	23	24	26	27	29	30	32	33	35	36
6'0"	16	18	19	20	22	23	24	26	27	28	30	31	33	34
6'2"	15	17	18	19	21	22	23	24	26	27	28	30	31	32
6'4"	15	16	17	18	20	21	22	23	24	26	27	28	29	30
6'6"	14	15	16	17	19	20	21	22	23	24	25	27	28	29
6'8"	13	14	15	17	18	19	20	21	22	23	24	25	26	28

Height in feet and inches

Underweight   Healthy weight   Overweight   Obese

© Infobase Publishing

Figure 1.2 Body Mass Index (BMI) is a commonly used guideline for determining the appropriateness of a person's weight based on his or her height.

the amount of body fat differs between girls and boys. To be considered overweight, a child or teen would be in the ninety-fifth percentile or higher for his or her age based on BMI. Being in the ninety-fifth percentile, for example, means that the individual's BMI is greater than 95 percent of the other individuals in the same age category. A child or teen in the eighty-fifth to ninety-fifth percentile is considered at risk for overweight, according to the Centers for Disease Control. The CDC does not provide a definition for obese children and teens, although the term childhood obesity is used in their literature.

In the United States, one-third of all adults are overweight, a statistic that has been consistent since 2002; the percentage of overweight children, however, is on the rise. According to the Mayo Clinic, since the 1980s, the prevalence of overweight children ages 6 to 11 doubled and the number of overweight teens tripled. According to the Centers for Disease Control, approximately 18.8 percent of U.S. children and 17.1 percent of teens are overweight. Being an overweight child or teen greatly increases the chances that he or she will be an overweight adult and therefore be at a greater risk for obesity-related health disorders, such as type 2 diabetes and heart disease.

The U.S. Food and Drug Administration (FDA) is the agency responsible for protecting the public from unsafe drugs; however, the FDA has much more control over prescription drugs than it does over nonprescription drugs and **dietary supplements**. A dietary supplement is a pill, capsule, powder, or liquid that supplies nutrients such as vitamins or minerals. A multivitamin is an example of a dietary supplement. Taking fish oil to assist with lowering blood cholesterol would be one way that a person might use a dietary supplement. Although the nutrients in supplements are in foods, the FDA does not consider them foods.

Drugs that require a prescription must produce research to show that they are safe and effective before the FDA approves them for sale. Dietary supplements do not have to be approved by the FDA to be sold. Dietary supplements must not, however, be marketed on false or misleading claims. The FDA can only intervene after the product has reached the market and there is evidence that it is dangerous to human health. This lack of regulation has proven to be a danger to the public, as is the case with ephedra, which caused several deaths before the FDA stepped in and banned this supplement.

2

Fat and Weight Loss

Mary is a 35-year-old mother of two daughters. Although she has always struggled with weight, her weight has hit an all-time high in the past few months. A couple of years ago, she injured her back, which left her unable to work. It was after her injury that she really started to gain weight, reaching more than 350 pounds. She considered back surgery but the doctor told her the risks were too great due to her weight-related health issues. Mary looked into getting her stomach stapled, hoping that she would lose enough weight to allow her to have the back surgery. However, her insurance would not pay for the surgery.

At her weight and with her back problems, Mary feels like she cannot exercise, creating a vicious cycle of weight gain and inactivity. Mary is just one of the 9 million Americans who are morbidly obese. If Mary continues to be morbidly obese she will likely suffer dozens of ailments from arthritis to asthma, and have her life shortened by 20 years. Weight-loss drugs, however, are often covered by insurance; if Mary tries them and is able to reduce her weight by 10 percent, she might become a better candidate for the back surgery she needs.

CHILDHOOD OBESITY

The rise in childhood obesity is believed to be due to increases in poor nutrition and inactivity. Television, computers, and other electronics are more popular with children today but generally offer no physical exercise. National guidelines recommend 150 minutes of physical activity per week for elementary school–age children and 225 minutes per week for older children and teens. In one survey completed by the Centers for Disease Control, 27.8 percent of high school girls and 43.8 percent of high school boys reported at least 60 minutes of exercise at least five times per week. High school boys are more likely than girls to be active because they are more likely to participate in sports. According to researchers at the University of South Carolina, one-third of teens are unfit, based on a study of more than 3,000 teens from 1999 to 2002. The definition of "unfit" was determined by a treadmill test where the teens' heart rates were monitored. The researchers found that overweight teens are much more likely to fail the fitness test than normal-weight teens and that boys are slightly more likely to meet the fitness standard than girls. The findings were troubling to medical professionals because it is well accepted that unfit teens are much more likely to be unfit adults.

Fast food and vending machines in schools also contribute to childhood obesity. For many children, fast food is a weekly or even daily part of their diets. Particularly disturbing is the quantity of sugar children consume today. According to the United States Department of Agriculture, in the early 1800s, the average person consumed approximately 12 pounds of sugar annually. By the 1970s, the annual consumption of sugar jumped to 137 pounds, a figure that has not changed much over the years despite the introduction of many artificial sweeteners. The source of much of this sugar is in **processed foods** and sweetened drinks.

Processed foods are foods made with processed white sugar, **high-fructose corn syrup**, and grains such as white flour, in which the plant fiber—and most of the nutrition—has been removed. High-fructose corn syrup (HFCS) is a sweetener created from corn syrup. Most "convenience" foods are processed. The danger with processed foods is that without fiber to slow the absorption of food, the glucose (sugar) from the broken-down food floods the bloodstream, causing the body to produce **insulin** to handle this excess sugar. The insulin captures the sugar, which may leave the person feeling

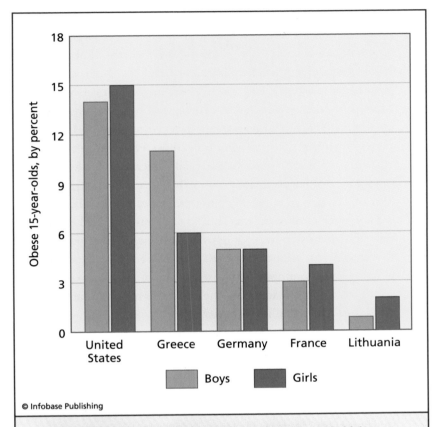

Figure 2.1 The United States' teenage obesity rate is higher than that of 14 other industrialized countries, some of which are shown in this graph. Experts say that the greater consumption of fast food in the United States contributes to this statistic. It is estimated that between 50 and 80 percent of obese teenagers will become obese adults.

tired and cranky from a suddenly lower blood sugar level. This cycle is commonly known as a sugar crash, and from a medical perspective is an unhealthy eating style. Having insulin levels fluctuate greatly as a result of a poor diet can increase the chances of developing type 2 diabetes.

Becoming overweight as a child can make weight loss a more significant struggle throughout life. Scientists identified adolescence as a critical period for the development of obesity. A person who becomes overweight during adolescence is much more likely to struggle with obesity later in life. An overweight adolescent has a greater chance of being obese as an adult than an overweight child who has not reached adolescence. The reason for this is that weight gain in adolescence increases the amount and size of fat cells. Once fat cells are created, they cannot be lost through weight loss. When an adolescent tries to lose weight, he or she can only limit the size of the fat cells and not the total number of fat cells. The only way to get rid of fat cells permanently is through liposuction, a surgical procedure in which the fat cells are removed from the body. Liposuction is not a realistic option for most people, so the best way to control adult obesity is to limit the proliferation of new fat cells developed from childhood obesity.

TYPE 2 DIABETES

Type 2 diabetes was previously referred to as adult-onset diabetes, whereas type 1 was referred to as juvenile diabetes. However, the onset of type 2 diabetes is occurring increasingly in younger people and is now seen in preteens. The statistics of young people developing what was once considered an adult disease is alarming. According to the Institute of Medicine, for children born in the United States in 2000, the lifetime risk of being diagnosed with type 2 diabetes is estimated at about 30 percent for boys and 40 percent for girls. Because type 2 diabetes has become a disease with childhood or adult onset, it is now referred to as noninsulin-dependent diabetes.

Type 2 diabetes is considered a preventable disease. The main difference between type 1 and type 2 is that type 2 diabetes is a reflection of a person's lifelong dietary habits. People with type 1 diabetes generally have a genetic tendency to develop the disease even if there is not a family history of diabetes. Environmental conditions such as exposure to a virus can also trigger diabetes in susceptible individuals. Risk factors for type 2 diabetes include a family history, age, and race. Family members of people with type 2 diabetes are at an increased risk of developing the disease. Likewise, as one ages, the chances of developing type 2 increase. For uncertain reasons, African Americans, American Indians, and Asian

IS IT RUDE TO REFER TO CHILDREN AS OBESE?

The National Association to Advance Fat Acceptance (NAAFA) believes that children should not be referred to as obese by the medical industry, government, or anybody else. NAAFA believes that referring to children as obese creates an environment in which children feel shame about their bodies. According to NAAFA, the stigmatization of large children has increased over the last 30 years. In fact, overweight children are more likely to be both victims and perpetrators of bullying, according to a study published in the journal *Pediatrics*. Obese children were more than twice as likely to be intentionally left out of social activities as their normal-weight peers. When obese children were asked to rate their quality of life, they ranked their happiness as low as young cancer patients, reportedly because of teasing and weight-related health problems.

NAAFA would prefer to embrace a variety of body types, even those that are larger, while encouraging healthy eating and physical activity. Medical professionals use the statistics about stigmatizing obese children and the emotional damage it is likely to cause as an additional reason to encourage weight loss. No one knows for sure whether removing the label of obese when referring to an obese child will make the child feel more comfortable with his or her body, but the issue can raise sensitivity about the stigmatization these children are likely to experience.

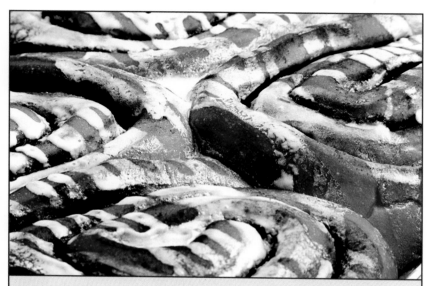

Figure 2.2 Processed foods are made with ingredients including white flour and white sugar. These foods, such as the cinnamon buns here, cause wide fluctuations in insulin and blood sugar levels, which lead to "sugar highs" and "sugar crashes," and contribute to the development of type 2 diabetes. (© Robert Gubbins/Shutterstock)

Americans are more likely to develop type 2 diabetes than Americans of European descent.

Although there is much that scientists do not understand about this disease, it is clear that weight and physical activity play a role. The more fatty tissue that a person has, the more resistant his or her body's cells will be to insulin. Being sedentary is also a risk factor. Physical activity not only controls weight but also helps to burn glucose and is believed to help the body be more sensitive to insulin.

To understand best how obesity and type 2 diabetes are linked, it is important to understand how glucose works in the body. Glucose is the source of energy for the body's cells and comes primarily from food. After eating, insulin, which is a hormone, is released from the pancreas into the blood-stream. Insulin is like a gatekeeper for the sugar to get into the cells. Without insulin, the bloodstream could be full of sugar but a person's cells could not access it and he or she would feel lethargic. In a properly working pancreas, insulin levels decrease in response to a drop in blood sugar levels. When the blood sugar dips too low, perhaps because too much time has elapsed since the last meal, the liver releases stored glucose to keep glucose levels at the appropriate range. For people with type 2 diabetes, this careful balancing act does not work properly, resulting in a buildup of glucose in the bloodstream or a potentially fatal situation if the blood glucose falls too low.

Type 2 diabetes is a condition in which the pancreas does not produce enough insulin to regulate the body's blood sugar level. If the blood sugar is not kept in control, this excess blood sugar may deposit in areas of the body and cause severe long-term consequences. People with diabetes are more prone to heart disease, blindness, kidney damage, and nerve damage.

This nerve damage is referred to as **diabetic neuropathy**. Diabetic neuropathy can cause tingling or even the loss of feeling in arms, feet, or any part of the body. This loss of feeling can enable cuts to go unnoticed, which can lead to infections. These infections can become so severe that amputation is the only treatment. Diabetic neuropathy is more common among diabetics who have had diabetes for more than 25 years, those who are overweight, and those who have poorly controlled blood sugar levels. In addition to neuropathy, type 2 diabetes also increases a person's risk of heart disease, blindness, and kidney damage.

OTHER HEALTH IMPLICATIONS

In addition to diabetes, obesity is linked to heart disease, **osteoarthritis** (pain in the joints as a result of abnormal wearing of the cartilage), high blood pressure, stroke, gallbladder disease, respiratory problems, and an increased risk of some kinds of cancer such as uterine, breast, and colon cancer. In a 2008 study by the Kaiser Permanente Division of Research in Oakland, California, researchers found a greater incidence of dementia linked with a potbelly, otherwise known as having an apple-shaped body type. In the study, the belly was measured using a set of calipers that measured from the back to the top of the abdomen. Those individuals measuring 10 inches from back to upper abdomen were classified to have an apple-shaped body. Researchers followed up on these individuals an average of 36 years later and found that the individuals with high belly measurements and normal weight were 89 percent more likely to have dementia than people

HIGH-FRUCTOSE CORN SYRUP: SWEET POISON?

All sugars are not broken down in the body in the same way. Research from Rutgers University in 2007 showed that high-fructose corn syrup (HFCS), the most common sweetener in sugary drinks and processed foods, might contribute to the nation's increase in type 2 diabetes.

High-fructose corn syrup does not occur naturally in any foods; it was created in the 1970s as an inexpensive substitute for sugar. Examining the label of many snacks and drinks will reveal HFCS as one of the first few ingredients—which indicates that it is present in greater proportion than ingredients farther down the list.

The biggest health concern is that HFCS contains high levels of highly reactive carbonyls. Chemicals with carbonyl groups are unstable and therefore likely to react with other molecules. Carbonyls, which are present in high levels in the blood of diabetics, are believed to cause tissue damage. Sugar is a more stable molecule and therefore does not produce carbonyls. Limiting the intake of sweeteners is always optimal; when offering sweetened food, parents should check labels and opt for sugar instead of HFCS.

with low belly measurements and normal body weight. Overweight people were 82 percent more likely to have dementia even if they had a low belly measurement and obese people with a low belly measurement were 81 percent more likely to develop dementia than their thinner counterparts. The researchers could not pinpoint exactly why the distribution of fat, not just a higher amount of body fat, would contribute to dementia but did theorize that the abdominal fat likely pumps out substances that harm the brain.[1]

Another disadvantage of having too much sugar in the bloodstream is repeated inflammation. Inflammation in

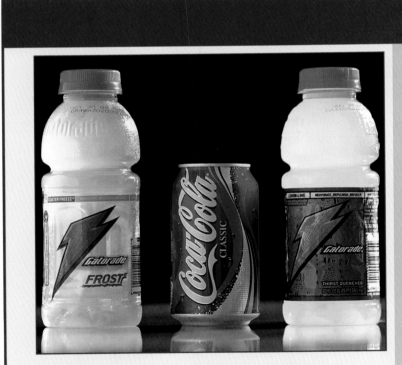

Figure 2.3 Sweetened soft drinks contain high-fructose corn syrup, an inexpensive alternative to sugar that was developed in the 1970s. (© Mike Blake/Reuters/Corbis)

the body is generally associated with infection. The red area around a cut is inflammation, caused by the rush of immune cells combating harmful bacteria that is trying to get into the body. The reddened area will eventually heal and then the redness goes away. A limited amount of inflammation such as this is unlikely to do damage but **chronic** inflammation can eventually cause tissue damage. Chronic indicates that the inflammation is persistent and ongoing. Too much glucose in the bloodstream can cause inflammation in the body, specifically in the heart.

The degree to which a person must be overweight to suffer from these obesity-related problems is debatable. Clearly those closer to the morbidly obese range have a much greater chance of developing these health problems than someone who has a mere 20 or 30 pounds to lose. A hotly debated 2007 study by the Centers for Disease Control and Prevention in Atlanta, Georgia, showed that people with a BMI between 25 and 30, which is considered overweight but not obese, have a lower death rate than people in the so-called normal, underweight, or obese weight ranges.[2] The researchers examined death records for 37,000 adults, along with age and weight to determine an individual's BMI. These records were then used to track trends in death rates with BMI. This study also found that being overweight did not increase the risk of dying from heart disease or cancer. Perhaps most surprisingly, the data indicated that the overweight were less likely die from other diseases such as chronic respiratory disease, Alzheimer's, infections, and Parkinson's. The researchers theorized that perhaps this excess fat served as an extra reserve during periods of illness. This study challenges the traditional notion that being overweight is unhealthy and leads to obesity-related health problems. The obese did not fare as well in this study, however. When researchers looked at the death records of people with BMIs ranking them as obese, they found that this group was at a higher risk for the diseases commonly associated with obesity.

This study has outraged many medical professionals such as Walter Willett, MD, professor of epidemiology and nutrition at the Harvard School of Public Health, who believes the findings should be completely disregarded. He argues that other studies have shown that being overweight can shorten one's life. Other critics say that the study does not address quality of life. These overweight individuals may not have died from their excess weight, but they may have suffered along the way, with osteoarthritis, for example. Most experts agree that tracking the impact of excess weight over a person's lifetime is difficult, and that it is particularly difficult to determine at which point certain illnesses or even death can be attributed to excess weight. It is important to realize that this is the first time in history that humankind has had such a prevalence of overweight and obese individuals, and therefore there is no clear data of exactly how this health factor affects death rates.

METABOLISM

Metabolism is the body's process of creating and using energy to support functions such as breathing and digesting. Because we cannot create our own energy from the Sun like plants can, we need to consume food to get energy. If our bodies were not constantly metabolizing food, then we could no longer live. Metabolism involves many complex chemical reactions in the body that enable a person to get a certain amount of energy—measured in calories—from eating an apple or even more energy from a slice of pizza.

Unused energy is stored in the body as fat. Energy reserves are a great survival mechanism, particularly in the days when famine was a threat. In the United States, scarcity of food is no longer a serious threat to survival so people do not have an opportunity to burn these energy reserves or fat. Americans also lead much more sedentary lives than people once did, often going from car to office cubicle with little physical exertion. In contrast, a pioneer who was chopping wood for hours a day would have much less chance of being overweight given the pioneer's high caloric needs. The abundance of food and reduced physical exertion in the average American's life has contributed significantly to the problem of obesity in the United States.

The metabolism rates of people vary, which plays a significant role in who will struggle with weight even if eating well and exercising. As a person ages, his or her metabolism will slow down, which contributes to weight gain in older years. Occasionally you will hear people mention that their weight gain is from a thyroid problem. A problem with this gland can definitely affect a person's weight. The thyroid gland produces a hormone called thyroxine, which affects the speed of metabolism. If the thyroid is damaged, it may become less active with the result of lowered metabolism. This condition is referred to as hypothyroidism. Individuals with hypothyroidism feel tired, feel constipated, and may have a slower heart rate. The opposite scenario is hyperthyroidism, when the thyroid is too active. The result of an overactive thyroid is weight loss, increased blood pressure, elevated heart rate, protruding eyes, and sometimes even a swelling of the neck referred to as a goiter.

Another factor affecting someone's metabolism is how much muscle he or she has and how much he or she exercises. Generally, a higher percentage of muscle versus fat on the body increases the metabolism. Exercise can increase metabolism because the body is burning more calories while running, jumping, or walking than while sitting still. The rate at which a person burns calories by sitting still is referred to as basal metabolism. Basal metabolism varies among people and is greatly influenced by genetics. Basal metabolism can be increased by becoming more physically fit. Another way to increase basal metabolism is by taking weight-loss drugs that stimulate the body's metabolic rate.

LIFESTYLE AND GENETICS

Diet, exercise, and genetics clearly play a pivotal role in weight. If obesity seems to run in the family, a struggle with weight could be the result of the genes a person inherited. According to the director of the Genomic Laboratory at Laval University Research Center in Quebec, Canada, an estimated 50 percent of obesity cases are due to genes. Currently, there are seven known gene defects that cause obesity.[3] A **gene defect** is a general term for a gene that causes the body to operate in an undesirable way, generally leading to disease. In this case, a gene defect could contribute to obesity, which then leads to heart disease.

Genetics cannot be controlled, but lifestyle can. One lifestyle choice is the hours of sleep a person gets each day. Sleep can factor into one's weight. **Leptin** is a hormone produced in the fat cells that signals to the brain that the body has had enough to eat. It is produced in relation to how much you sleep. Not getting enough sleep can drive down leptin levels. This drop in leptin level in turn can lead to overeating because the brain is not receiving the "full" signal. Another hormone that is affected by sleep is **ghrelin**. Ghrelin is a hormone produced in the gastrointestinal tract that stimulates appetite. Once food enters the stomach, the body halts ghrelin production. A lack of sleep can cause ghrelin levels to rise, leading to an increased sense of hunger. In essence, a chronic lack of sleep can cause a person to want to eat more and feel less satisfied than he or she would otherwise be when well rested.

Studies by the University of Chicago looked at this relationship between appetite and sleep. The researchers measured levels of leptin and ghrelin in 12 men. After those levels were measured the men were subjected to sleep deprivation for two days. Their levels were measured again. Then they received two days of extended sleep and again these hormone levels were measured. This experiment showed that leptin levels went down and ghrelin levels rose when sleep was restricted. The men also indicated that their appetite increased: Specifically, their desire for high-carbohydrate, calorie-dense foods increased by 45 percent.[4] This study shows that sleep deprivation may trigger the appetite and increase the likelihood of weight gain. Sleep, however, is just one of the lifestyle factors that affect one's weight; stress, dietary habits, and level of exercise also contribute significantly.

DIET AND EXERCISE

Diet and exercise are two of the most influential factors in weight loss. The term "diet" in this book is meant to refer to the day-to-day foods that a person generally chooses. It is the daily habits of food choices that have a stronger influence on weight management than the occasional overindulgence. For those who struggle with weight, they will need to restrict the overall amount of high-calorie foods they eat. Being too restrictive, however, can set up a person to fail at eating healthy. Often people become bored and feel deprived if certain groups of food, such as carbohydrates, are kept off limits. The diets with the best chance of success are those that are well balanced and do not demonize any specific foods. Many people evaluate a diet based on how quickly they can lose weight, but the best plans are actually those with which a person can comply long term.

One of the biggest challenges children face is that they often must eat the foods presented to them. One example would be school lunches. If a school cafeteria is only selling pizza, fries, and cheeseburgers, then the child without a packed lunch is at an immediate disadvantage for controlling calories. Luckily, some schoolchildren are getting the message that diet is crucial to maintaining health and proper weight. A group of five male students from Maple Point Middle School in Langhorne, Pennsylvania, desired a healthier option at lunchtime. With the help of their families, they petitioned the school to provide a salad bar. The new salad bar has fresh lettuce, low-fat dressing, and toppings such as chicken, tuna, oranges, cheese, tomatoes, croutons, eggs, and cucumbers. The school sold approximately a week's worth of lettuce within the first day of the salad bar's debut. A change in diet such as a hearty salad rather than a cheeseburger can help tremendously in maintaining a healthy weight.

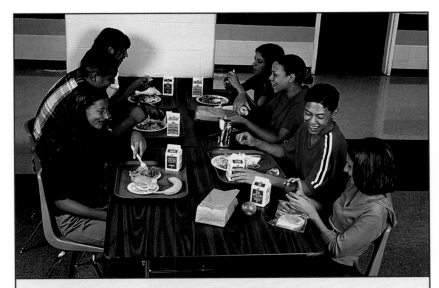

Figure 2.4 In an effort to reduce obesity in children and teen-agers, many school districts now offer healthy lunch options, such as salads, fresh fruits, and skim milk. (© Aaron Haupt/Photo Researchers, Inc.)

HEALTHY WEIGHT LOSS

A statistic often quoted in dieting literature is that 95 percent of people who lose weight gain it all back. According to the American Obesity Association, this statistic is no longer true and reflects a small study completed in 1959. Losing weight is not easy, but a person who commits to a plan of physical activity and moderate dieting will see results. Most importantly, it is necessary to replace poor dietary habits with good eating habits and exercise in order for the weight to stay off permanently.

Dieting for children who are still growing should be viewed with extreme caution. Children use their calories to develop, unlike adults, and too severe of a caloric restriction could impair this growth. According to the Mayo Clinic, if a child is

(continues on page 34)

MEASURING FAT: THE SKIN-FOLD TEST

Another method of evaluating a person's weight is estimating the percentage of body fat. Obese is defined as 32 percent or higher for women and 25 percent or higher for men. The amount of body fat a person has is nearly impossible to measure directly; many tests have been developed to estimate it. Many of these methods estimate body fat percentage by evaluating the density of a person's body by submerging him or her in water. Since fat is less dense then muscle and bone, formulas can be used that incorporate how much water a person has displaced to estimate his or her body fat percentage.

An easier, yet probably less accurate, way to estimate body fat percentage is a skin-fold test: Calipers measure the thickness of fat on various areas of the body. The calipers, which resemble tongs, are used to pinch typically fatty areas such as the stomach, thigh, or back of the upper arm. The measurements are then plugged into a formula to convert the thickness of these fat folds into a percentage of body fat. The numbers can fluctuate, however, depending on the type of calipers used, the consistency of the measurer, the distribution of body fat of the person being measured, and the formula used. The estimate is also dependent on the measurer testing in a precise location and using a fixed pressure. A measurer who presses too hard would increase the amount of fat measured and overestimate the fat percentage. The number of measurements taken can also affect the body fat estimate. Some formulas rely on seven measurements from the body, whereas other formulas only require three measurements. If a person is measured on the part of the body that is more fatty than other areas that are not measured, that individual's fat percentage could be overestimated. At best, these percentages might be used to measure the change in one person over a period of time if the same measurer and same areas of the body are used. As with all calculations used to determine the appropriateness of one's weight, the numbers do not take into account the variations in body type.

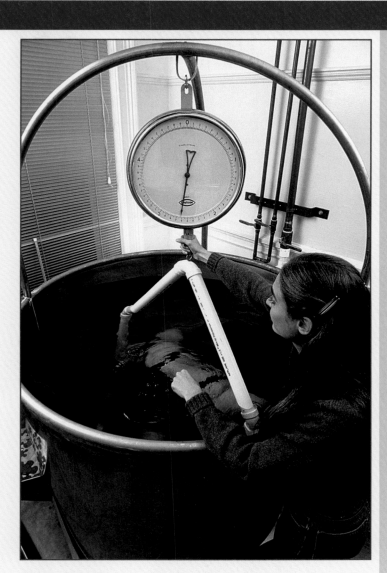

Figure 2.5 By submerging a person in water, his or her body fat percentage can be estimated. This calculation is based on how much water is displaced by a person and on the knowledge that muscle and bone are more dense than fat. (© Yoav Levy/ Phototake)

(continued from page 31)

overweight, weight loss is typically recommended if he or she is more than 7 years old. For overweight children younger than 7, weight maintenance is the goal. Younger overweight children who maintain their weight will actually be slimming down as they gain height, so their BMI will decrease. One general rule is true for any healthy weight loss: A slow and consistent weight loss is best, generally one pound per week.

A child's weight loss also greatly depends on the habits and eating attitudes of the adults in the home. When buying food for meals at home and school lunches, parents should shop primarily in the outer aisles of the supermarket; this is where stores stock fresh foods such as fruits, vegetables, and dairy products. Sitting down to eat as a family has also been shown to encourage more healthy eating because people sitting at a table rather than in front of the television are generally more aware of their food portions. Parents who limit the number of times the family eats out, particularly for fast food, will improve their child's nutrition. Parents who prepare their children's food at home are better able to control the portion size and ingredients. It has been well documented that restaurants have been increasing portion sizes, which has contributed to the obesity epidemic.

WEIGHT LOSS AND THE PLATEAU EFFECT

Anyone who has struggled with weight agrees that it seems much easier to gain weight than to lose it. A resistance to lose weight, even when we have excess fat, is scientifically proven.

Our bodies are programmed to gain weight when food intake increases (or exercise decreases) and resist weight loss when food seems to become scarce. This mechanism was developed as a survival technique in times of famine. When food intake suddenly diminishes, the body assumes that food supply is scarce and protects the individual's survival by resisting weight loss. The body has no way of knowing that a refrigerator full of food is just steps away. The resistance to lose weight can often increase after a couple months of dieting. A person may lose a pound per week for a couple months on a healthy diet and exercise routine but then stop seeing results while still maintaining this regimen. This leveling off of weight loss is known as the **plateau effect**. Health professionals recommend increasing the intensity or duration of physical activity to fight the body's determination to keep that extra fat. On the other hand, the plateau effect is a great incentive not to gain too much excess weight in the first place.

3

Appetite Suppressants

Most of the current weight-loss drugs approved by the FDA are appetite suppressants. Appetite suppressants aid weight loss in one of three ways. One approach is to reduce appetite by blocking the part of the brain that makes you crave food. The second way is to stimulate the part of the brain that makes you feel full to the point of being satisfied, also known as being satiated. A third approach is to slow down stomach emptying, causing a person to feel more full with less food. The appetite can be suppressed by altering brain chemistry, such as by increasing levels of **serotonin**. Serotonin is a chemical that creates a feeling of satisfaction in the body.

THE APPETITE CENTER: HYPOTHALAMUS

The desire to eat, or appetite, is controlled by the appetite center of the brain, also known as the **hypothalamus**. The hypothalamus is influenced by a complex interaction of hormones, the digestive tract, and the nervous system. If a person's stomach is empty, the blood sugar level decreases, and a message goes to the hypothalamus. When a person's blood sugar is low, serotonin levels may also be low, and in addition to feeling hungry a person could feel irritable and have a heightened craving for foods that release serotonin, including foods high in carbohydrates. Foods high in carbohydrates include cake, cookies, and crackers that quickly break down into sugar available to the body for energy.

As a result of low blood sugar levels and low serotonin, the hypothalamus is stimulated and a person feels hunger. Once a person has eaten enough, serotonin is produced, which creates a feeling of being full instead of a feeling of hunger. An individual can easily associate a late afternoon slice of cake with these increased levels of serotonin and develop a habit that is difficult to break.

Stress, hormones, and depression also affect levels of chemicals in the body, such as serotonin, thus triggering the desire to eat. Some researchers, such as Dr. Judith Wurman, author of *Managing Your Mind and Mood Through Food,* believe that many obese people treat their "blah" feelings by indulging in carbohydrate-rich foods that boost their serotonin levels and therefore improve their mood, at least temporarily. This pattern of seeking out foods rich in carbohydrates to treat "blah" feelings often leaves the individual feeling worse as the body floods the bloodstream with insulin and blood sugar levels dip, also know as a "sugar crash." Despite the resulting sugar crash, the pursuit of carbohydrate-rich foods is a difficult habit to break for a person trying to boost his or her mood through food. The relationship between cravings and serotonin levels encouraged the use of drugs, such as sibutramine, which boost serotonin levels to promote weight loss.

Appetite, however, is not strictly driven by the quantity and timing of the most recent meal. A change in hormones, for example, such as those associated with pregnancy, could increase appetite. Illness or stress could cause a decrease or increase in appetite. Cortisol is a hormone that is secreted under stress. Women with higher levels of cortisol have been found in research experiments to snack on higher-fat foods than those with lower cortisol levels. Cortisol is just one example of a hormone released by the body that influences eating habits.

One way to control the desire to eat is to alter the signaling system in the brain that stimulates appetite. **Neurotransmitters** are chemicals in the brain that carry messages between the brain's **neurons**. In the case of the neurotransmitter serotonin, this signaling system lets the body know it is full or hungry.

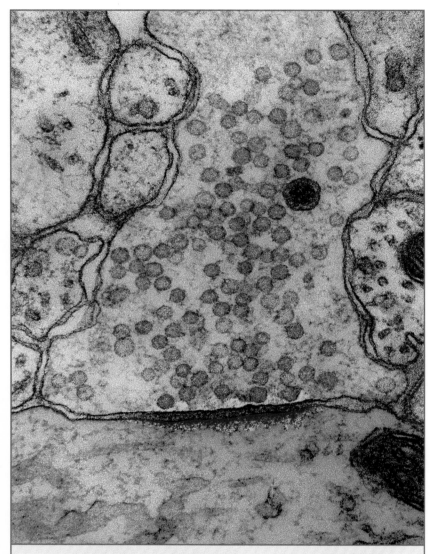

Figure 3.1 This transmission electron microscope image (TEM) shows neurotransmitters (purple dots) moving between two neurons (pink and green areas) in the brain. Some weight-loss drugs stimulate the production of the neurotransmitter serotonin, which signals to the body that it is full. (© Dr. Dennis Kunkel/Visuals Unlimited, Inc.)

AMPHETAMINES AND APPETITE SUPPRESSANTS

The currently FDA-approved appetite suppressants belong to a group of drugs called phenethylamines, which are similar to **amphetamines**. Amphetamines are known to have a stimulant effect on the **central nervous system**. Central nervous system (CNS) stimulants are drugs that can speed up mental or physical functions. One of the most common CNS stimulants is caffeine.

The appetite suppressants discussed in this section are CNS stimulants. The way that these drugs control appetite is by stimulating the part of the brain that controls appetite. As mentioned, the hypothalamus is the appetite center of the brain so it makes sense that a group of drugs that controls appetite would influence the brain.

These CNS stimulants affect a number of neurotransmitter systems in the brain, including serotonin. For those with weight problems, taking a pill to stave off hunger may seem like magic. However, altering chemicals in the body, even by adding a "feel-good" hormone such as serotonin, has risks as well as benefits. Although scientific results show an increase in weight loss as compared with a **placebo** or no pill, the weight loss is minimal: a fraction of a pound per week. For some, this small amount of weight loss due to the drug makes it worthwhile, especially when they factor in the mental and physical toll of obesity; for others, the side effects outweigh the benefits.

CNS stimulants also have side effects that pose a risk to the consumers. These stimulants increase the heart rate and blood pressure and therefore might not be recommended for people with high blood pressure or heart problems. Side effects vary but often include insomnia, irritability, and nervousness. The same drug could cause different reactions, so one person might experience a side effect that another patient taking the same drug may not. Some consumers find that the short-term side effects are simply not worth the weight loss. Others may not experience these side effects but could, in later years, encounter long-term side effects that are currently unknown. The research on side effects involves only short-term experiments so it is difficult to know for sure what long-term side effects could occur.

Phentermine

Phentermine is an appetite suppressant that was approved by the FDA in 1959 for short-term treatment of obesity. Phentermine stimulates a group of neurotransmitters known as catecholamines, which signal a flight-or-fight response in the body. It is believed that the brain does not receive the hunger signal because it is receiving the fight-or-flight signal and focusing on the immediate need for energy. It is also believed that phentermine increases the level of the hormone leptin, which signals the body to feel full.

In addition to increasing hormones that make a person feel full, phentermine also inhibits another neurotransmitter, neuropeptide Y. This neurotransmitter signals the body to eat, decrease physical activity, and increase fat storage. The combination of making a person feel full, increasing the desire to be more physically active, and inhibiting hunger and fat storage made phentermine seem like a great combination.

Like many of the first weight-loss drugs, phentermine is meant for short-term use, generally no longer than six months. Most users of phentermine can expect to see one-half to one pound of weight loss per week. One study of 24 weeks showed that phentermine users lost 22 pounds compared to 10 pounds of weight loss by people receiving a placebo. During the experiment, all participants were given an individualized diet, which explains why the people taking the placebo lost weight.[1] The idea is that once a person gets a "jump start" on weight loss from the drug, he or she would feel motivated to maintain the loss or ideally lose more through diet and exercise. The long-term effects of phentermine are unknown.

Phentermine is most notorious for its potentially fatal interaction with two other weight-loss drugs, fenfluramine

(Fen-phen) and dexfenfluramine (Redux), which can cause a rare lung disorder called pulmonary hypertension as well as heart valve disease. When phentermine is used alone, however, this danger appears to be absent; for this reason, this drug continues to be sold under the brand names Adipex-P, Fastin, Obenix, Phentercot, Pro-Fast, and Teramine. Users of phentermine are warned by the manufacturer about this dangerous interaction with fenfluramine and dexfenfluramine.

Phendimetrazine

Phendimetrazine is also in the phenethylamine class of drug and is sold under the brand names Bontril, Plegine, Prelu-2, and X-Trozine. Phendimetrazine was approved by the FDA in 1976 and is meant for the first few weeks of a diet and exercise program for the obese.

Phendimetrazine stimulates the central nervous system, just as phentermine does, but it has more of a noticeable stimulating effect than does phentermine. Phendimetrazine is available as time-release capsules and as a result, patients report having more energy throughout the day, even when they are not active. Phendimetrazine does not have the same level of cravings control as phentermine. Phendimetrazine could be prescribed for the first few weeks of a diet to assist with initial weight loss, after which the patient could be prescribed phentermine to assist with continuing appetite control. Both of these drugs could play a role in an overall plan of weight reduction that includes diet and exercise.

Phendimetrazine can increase blood pressure and is therefore not recommended for people with high blood pressure. Other side effects include dizziness, insomnia, headache, dry mouth, and constipation. Phendimetrazine can also become habit forming if used beyond the recommended first few weeks of a diet. Used alone, phendimetrazine has not been reported to cause the same types of lung or heart valve problems that Fen-phen or Redux did. However, if phendimetrazine is combined with other appetite suppressants, specifically phentermine, or is used in higher than recommended doses or for too long, lung and heart valve problems may occur.

Diethylpropion

The FDA approved diethylpropion in 1959 for the short-term treatment of obesity, usually for just a few weeks because it can become habit forming. Diethylpropion is meant to be a supplement to a diet and exercise regimen. It is sold under the brand name Tenuate by Watson. Similar to the other appetite suppressants, diethylpropion is an amphetamine-like drug that stimulates the central nervous system.

In one study lasting 25 weeks, Tenuate decreased weight by 26 pounds compared to a loss of 3.5 pounds for placebo users on a diet. In another study of 12 weeks, Tenuate users lost 20 pounds and placebo users lost 10 pounds while on a highly restrictive diet of 1,000 calories.[2] A weight loss of more than one pound a week is not recommended. A diet of only 1,000 calories is also too restrictive even for someone on a diet, particularly if he or she is exercising.

The exact mechanism by which diethylpropion stimulates the central nervous system to suppress appetite is not well understood. Side effects include sleeplessness and nervousness. Diethylpropion can also become addictive if used long term. Because it is a stimulant, people with heart disease, high blood pressure, an overactive thyroid, or glaucoma should not use this drug. Although Tenuate has been in use since 1959, it is not a popular weight-loss drug choice.

Sibutramine

The FDA approved sibutramine, one of the more popular appetite suppressants made by Abbott Laboratories, in 1997. The brand names include Meridia in North America and Reductil in other countries.

Sibutramine is unique in that it is approved by the FDA for long-term use, which is likely the cause of its popularity. Although many appetite suppressants are used off label for longer than a few weeks or months, this is not considered to be an FDA-approved use. (Orlistat is another weight-loss drug approved by the FDA for long-term use.) The typical cost of a 30-day supply of Meridia is $112 to $213; however, many medical insurance plans might cover it because a patient cannot purchase this medication without a doctor's prescription.

Sibutramine works in the same manner as phentermine, by increasing levels of catecholamines and inhibiting neuropeptide Y, but sibutramine also increases levels of serotonin in the body. Sibutramine has been shown to cause at least 5 percent weight loss in 85 percent of obese patients and at least 10 percent weight loss in 57 percent of its consumers.[3] This drug has been associated with increased blood pressure, headaches, dry mouth, insomnia, and constipation, so people with a history of heart disease or stroke should not take it. People who take certain antidepressants that increase serotonin levels cannot take sibutramine because of the risk of serotonin toxicity.

OVER-THE-COUNTER APPETITE SUPPRESSANTS

Not all appetite suppressants require a prescription. Hundreds of products exist that claim to squelch hunger pangs. Do these products really work? Unlike prescription drugs, over-the-counter supplements do not need FDA approval and therefore do not have to prove that their products really work before they are sold. If people find that the claims are false once the product has been sold, the Federal Trade Commission (FTC) can intervene for false and misleading advertising. If the product is found to be dangerous, then the FDA can get involved and ban the product.

Purchasing over-the-counter appetite suppressants can be dangerous. The main danger is that people often take the new drug without consulting a doctor to learn about possible interactions with prescribed medications. Consumers might also erroneously follow the "more is better" motto and take more pills than is recommended. Whereas a prescription refill limit helps prevent such abuse, supplements can be purchased as frequently as the buyer wishes. Two of the most popular supplements are hoodia and 5-HTP, which can be purchased in health food stores and on the Internet. Many people are not concerned with the lack of regulation of these drugs that are derived from plants and therefore "natural," unlike prescription drugs, which are often synthetic. The distinction of a drug being natural because it is derived from a plant is not necessarily valid. In fact, some of the most lethal compounds come from plants!

HOODIA

Hoodia advertisements on the Internet are ubiquitous, many in the form of pop-ups that claim to melt away fat within days. With this type of glitzy advertising, one might consider the product worth a try. Unfortunately, legitimate scientific literature does not indicate if hoodia actually suppresses appetite and what kind of loss one can expect.

Hoodia is an ingredient found naturally in a cactus-like plant, *Hoodia gordonii*, which grows in the Kalahari Desert in southern Africa. Hoodia is one of the most popular over-the-counter diet pills today, but it has actually been used for decades. A Dutch anthropologist who observed the Bushmen of the Kalahari Desert first noted hoodia's supposed appetite-suppressing qualities in the early 1900s. The anthropologist noted that these nomadic people ate the stem of the hoodia plant to control their hunger while on long hunting trips where there was little vegetation to eat. According to Jan Vander Westhuitzen, a South African Bushman tracker, a sip of hoodia's bitter liquid gave people enough energy to walk all day.

A British pharmaceutical company, Phytopharm, researched the ingredients in hoodia and isolated the appetite-suppressing aspect of the plant to a molecule referred to as P57. The scientists from Phytopharm believe that P57 acts on the appetite center of the brain, making it think the body is full. Phytopharm sublicensed rights to another pharmaceutical

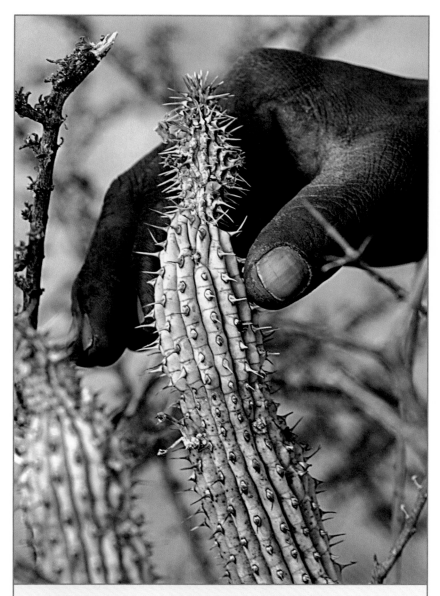

Figure 3.2 The hoodia cactus has been traditionally used by the San people in Africa to suppress appetite while on hunting trips. In recent years hoodia has become a popular dietary supplement in the West. This popularity has led to this plant becoming an endangered species. (© AP Images)

company, Pfizer, with intentions to use this extract from hoodia as a prescription weight-loss drug. Pfizer lost interest in pursuing P57 as a weight-loss drug after realizing that the molecule would be too difficult to synthesize and package in a pill. Phytopharm and another company, Unilever, are examining the feasibility of incorportating P57 into food and beverages.

If the hoodia is so difficult to synthesize, this raises the question of where the supplement companies get their hoodia, and more specifically, the part of the hoodia plant that contains P57. Harvesting the plant from the desert is one possibility. However, the popularity of hoodia has increased harvesting to the extent that the plant is now on the endangered species list. Some manufacturers indicate that they grow it on a farm, but how and where is not clear. Even Westhuitzen, the South African Bushman, said that hoodia is in trouble because the land where it grows has become too dry.

Unilever completed tests on 10 different supplement brands of hoodia and found that two contained no significant quantities of P57, four contained small amounts of it, and four others contained significant amounts.[4] It was not clear from the study what defined "a significant amount," but then again, no one really knows how much is needed to lose weight. There have not been any scientific studies on the effectiveness of hoodia or P57 alone to determine how much is needed and for how long to see a statistically significant weight loss. Hoodia's popularity is amazing in light of the fact that all success stories are purely anecdotal, meaning that people might talk about its effectiveness but there is no research to back up the claims.

No one has yet examined the safety of hoodia in humans. Early research by Pfizer indicated that P57 is broken down in the liver. This concerns some doctors because many obese people suffer from liver disease. When a person becomes overweight, the liver usually cannot handle the fat levels in the body and the fat becomes stored in the liver. As a result, the liver becomes enlarged and can become permanently scarred. An enlarged and scarred liver will not be able to function as well as a healthy liver. A weight-loss doctor in Oklahoma City, Dr. Michael Steelman, believes that the inadequate functioning of an obese person's liver could compound any side effect from hoodia. Nobody has determined what the side effects of taking hoodia might be, however, because researchers have yet to do studies on humans. Therefore, a user of hoodia would have to take his or her chances rather than rely on sound science.

Until the drug becomes regulated, users must take notice of their own side effects. Hoodia has been reported to cause many of the side effects associated with other appetite suppressants that act on the brain. These side effects include chest pain and migraines.[5]

5-HTP

5-Hydroxytryptophan, known as 5-HTP, is used as a supplement to control appetite. Like hoodia, 5-HTP is considered natural because it is an extract from the seed of an African shrub, *Griffonia simplicifolia* and because 5-HTP is the precursor to serotonin in the body. The theory is that if the precursor to serotonin is supplied externally, levels of serotonin will increase. It is for this reason that, in addition to its use as an appetite suppressant, 5-HTP has gained popularity with the health supplement industry for use in the treatment of ailments associated with low serotonin, including migraines, insomnia, depression, and chronic pain.

Manufacturers of 5-HTP supplements do not have any scientifically valid experiments proving their ability to control appetite or cause weight loss. Similar to other supplements, FDA control is very limited unless users suffer extreme health problems or die as a direct result of their use of 5-HTP. Consumers should be especially cautious if they have other risk factors, such as heart disease, or if they are taking other medication, such as antidepressants.

PPA (Phenylpropanolamine)

Since the 1970s, products that contain phenylpropanolamine, also known as PPA, have been available over the counter to control appetite under brand names such as Dexatrim and Acutrim. PPA was considered a drug and was regulated by the FDA. It was one of the only regulated weight-loss drugs that have been available without a prescription.

In November 2000, the FDA requested that manufacturers of products with PPA in them remove them from the market because a study showed that PPA increases the risk of hemorrhagic stroke. Hemorrhagic stroke is a condition where there is bleeding into the brain or into tissue surrounding the brain. PPA stimulates the central nervous system and causes an increased heart rate, just as prescription appetite suppressants do. Although the risk of hemorrhagic stroke due to PPA consumption was very rare, safer drugs to control appetite were available to consumers. The FDA found it difficult to predict who would be at risk of suffering a stroke as a result of taking PPA and decided to ban PPA in order to ensure that no one would experience this serious possible side effect.

This type of advisory shows the seriousness of taking any over-the-counter medications. Be sure to mention any over-the-counter drugs when asked by a medical professional what medications you take.

TEENS AND APPETITE SUPPRESSANTS

With the images of waifish women such as Nicole Richie, Victoria Beckham, Keira Knightley, and Mary-Kate Olsen in the pages of magazines, it is no wonder that teen girls use appetite suppressants to lose pounds. Consider Keira Knightley's BMI of 16.4, for example, which puts her in the underweight category. She is perceived by many as an object of male desire. Even comments posted on the Internet below an article about her near-starvation body weight (105 pounds at a height of 5'7") have readers posting comments such as "she's definitely too skinny, but she has fantastic abs. I would starve myself for

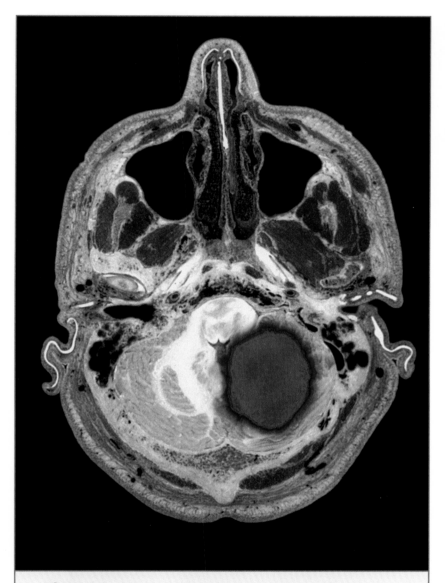

Figure 3.3 A hemorrhagic stroke occurs when a blood vessel bursts inside the brain. Here you can see that a stroke has happened on the right side of the person's brain (red). The diet drug PPA caused an elevated risk of hemorrhagic stroke and was eventually banned by the FDA. (© Scott Camazine/SPL/Custom Medical Stock Photo)

those!"[6] Brad Pitt, on the other hand, also considered quite attractive, has a BMI of 27, which is the average BMI for middle-aged American men. With these gender discrepancies among icons of beauty, it is no wonder that diet pills are much more a female issue than a male one.

A study completed in 2006 at the University of Minnesota found that the use of over-the-counter diet pills by high school–age females had nearly doubled over a five-year period, from 7.5 percent to 14.2 percent. Most doctors will not prescribe

THE TREND OF CLEN

Clenbuterol, commonly known as "clen," is a CNS stimulant that works by relaxing the muscles in the airways. It is used legally as an asthma treatment for horses, and many women in Hollywood are rumored to use it as a quick, although risky, weight-loss treatment. Although no celebrities admit to using the drug, some of the people who have allegedly used clen have been noted for their dramatic weight loss, going from a healthy weight to severely underweight with "chicken wing" arms, sagging breasts, gaunt faces, and bones protruding in the back. Some insiders refer to one well-known, clen-dispensing celebrity stylist as a "horse," and her stable of young, beautiful star clients as "mares."[7]

Similar to other CNS stimulants, clenbuterol suppresses appetite, speeds up the heart rate, and elevates blood pressure. It also helps burn fat and build muscle. Scientists do not fully understand how it can build muscle, but the stimulating aspects of clenbuterol produce the fat-burning capabilities of this drug. Many dieters consider clen superior to ephedrine because it stays in the body longer and does not affect sleep.

The safety of clenbuterol for human consumption has not been well studied. Most of the information about this drug pertains to animals, and the results of those animal studies weight-loss drugs to teens, particularly those with only mild weight issues. As a result, some teens might indiscriminately self-administer diet pills including hoodia, 5-HTP, and ephedra.

The teens surveyed in this University of Minnesota study who were taking diet pills were also found to engage in frequent unhealthy eating behaviors, such as skipping meals, using laxatives, and forcing themselves to vomit. In addition, the diet-pill-popping teens were three times more likely to be overweight.

raise concerns about human use. In rats, clenbuterol stiffens the heart, causing doctors to fear that clenbuterol use in humans could increase the risk of strokes and heart arrhythmia. In Europe, people cannot administer clenbuterol on any animal that will enter the food chain.

Despite the risks, it is easy to purchase clenbuterol over the Internet. A quick search on the Internet shows thousands of sites offering to sell clenbuterol and an equal number of postings exchanged by bodybuilders and dieters on how much to self-administer. One poster on a Web site called Clenbuterol King gives specifics about an accidental overdose: "My heart rate when I got to the emergency room was 178 and at its peak about two hours later just above 200."[8]

Even if a person does not accidentally overdose or damage his or her heart, using clen can permanently damage a user's metabolism. One user stated that she lost weight on clen but that the efficacy of the drug seemed to diminish quickly, because eating anything other than tuna fish caused her to "just blow up."[9] Interestingly, it is the potential for slowing the metabolism that has caused some hopeful dieters to hesitate before trying out clen. It is clear that for many trying to emulate the figures of Hollywood stars, heart damage pales compared to the fear of a slower metabolism.

When it comes to losing weight, any promotion of quick weight loss by the manufacturers of over-the-counter supplements should be regarded as junk science. These manufacturers do not have to provide solid, scientific evidence to the FDA and therefore generally do not have any legitimate studies to back up their claims. Luckily, there are ways to control appetite in healthy ways without the use of pills, patches, or teas.

THE ROLE OF WEIGHT-LOSS DRUGS IN GOOD HEALTH

Appetite suppressants do not offer a miracle cure for obesity. They all have their potential side effects from dry mouth to headaches, and the possibility for dependence if taken long term. Children under the age of 12 are advised not to use them.

These drugs are meant to act as an incentive for those beginning a weight-loss routine, enabling them to see more loss of pounds than dieting and exercise alone. These drugs, in a sense, are like a carrot dangled in front of a horse to get the animal moving in the right direction. The body can develop a resistance to appetite suppressants, so people who choose to integrate these drugs in a weight-loss plan must think about them as only short-term motivation. If a patient decides to use these drugs, he or she will also need to make major lifestyle changes to keep the unwanted pounds away permanently.

CONTROLLING APPETITE NATURALLY

The appetite can be controlled without taking drugs that alter brain chemistry. Eating water-dense fruits and vegetables such as apples, watermelons, and celery at the beginning of a meal, perhaps even allowing a bit of time for digestion, can help a person feel more full while consuming fewer calories. Drinking water throughout the day can also reduce hunger; in fact, a dehydrated person might mistake thirst for hunger pangs.

Drinking water also has the added benefit of slightly increasing the metabolism. Researchers in Berlin, Germany, found that their subjects had a 30 percent increase in metabolism after drinking approximately 17 ounces of water. The increases occurred within 10 minutes of drinking the water and the researchers estimate that up to 40 percent of the increase in calorie burning is from the body's attempt to heat the water. A person who consumes an additional 1.5 liters a day for a year could burn an additional 17,400 calories, which translates to a five-pound weight loss.[10]

Yet another way to maintain a modest appetite is to eat more, smaller meals. By eating more frequently, you will find that you feel less hungry at the next meal even if eating smaller portions. Eating more often also has the added benefit of boosting the metabolism while keeping blood sugar stabilized to avoid low blood sugar–induced fatigue, also known informally as a "sugar crash." When a person skips breakfast, the body has not received fuel in quite some time and may trick the body into "thinking" food is not plentiful. As a survival mechanism, the body's metabolism will slow down in order to preserve the calories from the previous night's dinner. As a result, people who eat breakfast are much more likely to weigh less, according to the National Weight Control Registry. A dieter should always be sure to eat breakfast to keep his or her metabolism revving and to resist the urge to indulge in bigger meals at lunch or dinner.

4

Lipase Inhibitors

Sandy is a fifteen-year-old girl spending the summer at camp, specifically a weight-loss camp. Sandy went to camp on her parents' insistence. She did not put up too much of a fight because, deep down, she hoped she might come back from camp as slim as her sisters. Even though Sandy ate the same foods as her parents and sisters, she seemed to have bulges in places that nobody else did. At least by going to camp, she would be around people who could understand her struggles. She felt positive about camp until it came time for the weekly weigh-ins and she had to step on the scale. Even while sticking to the lousy cafeteria food, Sandy just did not seem to be losing much weight. Sandy was at her wit's end until one of the other campers offered her some Alli. She vaguely remembered seeing a display in Target. Her fellow camper said it would definitely help her lose weight although she would be making more frequent trips to the outhouse. Sandy was willing to do anything and took the pills. Her friends and family back home knew she was going to "fat camp," as they called it, and she felt pressure to show results. Sandy felt bloated, crampy, and uncomfortable, but looked forward to the next weigh-in figuring all this discomfort had to pay off.

Lipase inhibitors reduce the body's ability to absorb fat, generally by one-third. These drugs are able to do this by blocking **lipase**, the enzyme that breaks down fat. Most of the fat consumed is passed through the body, which poses some undesirable side effects. Alli is one lipase inhibitor that can be purchased without a prescription.

CALORIES, CARBOHYDRATES, PROTEIN, AND FAT

Calories are measures of energy. Specifically, one calorie is the energy needed to increase the temperature of water by $1°C$. When one eats food, the body's digestion process releases this energy so that cells can use it. Higher-calorie foods require more energy to burn the energy they provide. Any unburned energy is stored as fat.

When a body burns energy, it usually burns fat and carbohydrates in a 50/50 split, assuming both are available in the body. Starchy foods such as breads, pastas, cereals, and potatoes are high in carbohydrates. Carbohydrates contain 4 calories per gram. Fat, on the other hand, has 9 calories per gram, which is why foods with a high fat content require more energy to burn: Those foods contain many more calories per gram than carbohydrates or even proteins, which have 4 calories per gram, just as carbohydrates do. Protein is found primarily in nuts, beans, soy, and meats.

The body needs fats, proteins, and carbohydrates to function properly. The United States Department of Agriculture (USDA) recommends proportions of each of these nutrients in the food pyramid. The USDA advises that people get 45 to 65 percent of daily calories from carbohydrates. Carbohydrates provide the main and most easily accessed source of energy for the body. Carbohydrates are stored in the muscles and liver. The kidneys, brain, and muscles (including the heart) all rely on carbohydrates to function properly.

Protein is needed in smaller quantities (10 to 35 percent of calories) than carbohydrates but is necessary for immune function, tissue repair, hormone and enzyme maintenance, and preserving and growing muscle mass. Protein is particularly vital for maintaining growth in children, teens, and pregnant women. Fats are recommended at 20 to 35 percent of total calories and are crucial for absorbing certain nutrients such as vitamins A, D, E, and K, as well as maintaining

The Food Pyramid

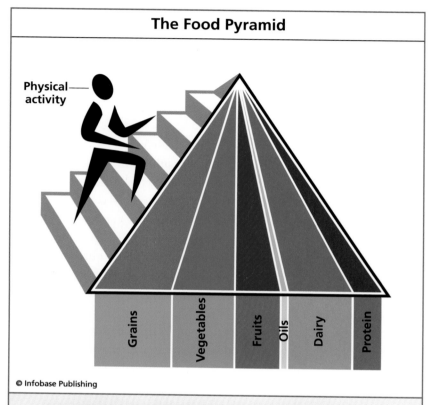

Physical activity

Grains Vegetables Fruits Oils Dairy Protein

© Infobase Publishing

Figure 4.1   In 2005 the USDA revised the food pyramid to incorporate its updated dietary guidelines. These new guidelines are customizable to fit different dietary lifestyles, such as vegetarian and vegan diets. The new food pyramid also recommends at least 30 minutes of physical activity each day. Individuals can calculate their dietary needs, based on factors such as age, sex, height, and activity level by visiting http://www.mypyramid.gov.

cell membranes. Fat enhances the taste and consistency of foods. A diet completely void of fat could leave your skin dry and hair brittle. In moderation, fat is an important part of a healthy diet.

Plenty of diets exist that manipulate the percentages of fat, carbohydrates, and proteins and pitch the equation as the remedy for obesity. The Atkins Diet, created by Dr. Robert Atkins, is a high-protein, low-carbohydrate program with percentages of calories from protein that are proportionally higher than the USDA recommends. The idea of this diet is that increasing protein and decreasing carbohydrates forces the body to burn fat while maintaining and encouraging muscle development. The Atkins Diet is more complex than the USDA's food pyramid and includes various phases, including carbohydrate intake changes and blood sugar monitoring to make sure that blood sugar is low enough so the body is forced to burn fat. This state where fat, instead of carbohydrates, is burned is known as **ketosis** and is a vital aspect of the Atkins Diet. Dieters in a state of ketosis will often have a metallic taste in their mouth or bad breath as a result of the body producing ketones, which is chemically similar to acetone or nail polish remover.

One reported disadvantage of this diet is that severely limiting carbohydrates reduces the amount of fiber in the diet. Fiber is found in whole grains, fruits, and vegetables. Fiber is the part of the carbohydrate that is not digested. Fiber has the critical role of moving waste out of the body, thus preventing constipation and hemorrhoids. Diets high in fiber decrease risks for heart disease and obesity, and help lower cholesterol. Another criticism of the Atkins Diet is that the amount of red meat in the diet increases the risk of heart disease. Most diets include meats that are lower in fat, such as fish and chicken. The Atkins Diet, however, does rightly link the consumption of refined foods with obesity. Although the Atkins Diet restricts the consumption of carbohydrates more than the USDA's food pyramid, Atkins makes a valid point that not all carbo-hydrates are equal when it comes to healthy eating and weight loss. Whole grains and fruits are much healthier carbohydrate choices than crackers and cookies made with bleached flour and high-fructose corn syrup.

Diets that restrict any one food group or nutrient are highly suspect and have a greater chance of failure because many

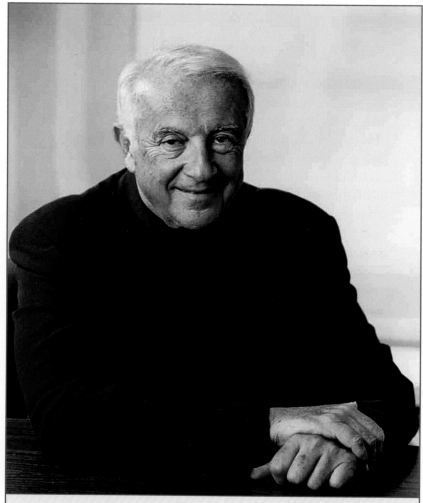

Figure 4.2 Dr. Robert Atkins, who devised the popular Atkins Diet. (© AP Images)

people may feel deprived and binge once their diet is over. It is also an unnecessary strategy for weight loss. If a person desires to lose weight, the USDA's food pyramid can assist with planning a healthy diet to achieve and maintain weight loss.

ENZYMES AND LIPASE

Enzymes are proteins that accelerate a chemical reaction without being consumed in the process. For example, enzymes in the stomach are able to break down food for digestion. Without these digestive enzymes, we would not be able to access many of the vitamins and minerals in our foods.

Lipase is an enzyme that breaks down fat in the body. It is produced in the pancreas and is not present in food. Lipase serves an important role because it enables the nutrients in fat to be broken down and absorbed in the intestines. A higher-fat meal would require more lipase to digest, whereas a low-fat meal would require less lipase. Without lipase, the fat, as well as any beneficial nutrients, cannot be absorbed by the body. This fat does not simply disappear; it passes through the intestines undigested, potentially with unsavory side effects.

ORLISTAT

Walk into a drugstore and you are likely to see a crisp white display with colorful lettering for orlistat under the trade name, Alli (pronounced "ally"). Alli is the first federally approved, over-the-counter weight-loss drug. Before Alli, orlistat was sold only by prescription by Roche under the brand name, Xenical; the FDA approved Xenical in 1999 for long-term use by obese patients. Alli is a lower dosage (60 milligrams) than the prescription Xenical (120 milligrams). Orlistat is also currently FDA approved for people who are 12 and older. Now that orlistat is available over the counter, however, it can be purchased by anyone, even those who are only slightly overweight or those who are not overweight but think they are.

Alli encourages weight loss by inhibiting lipase, thereby preventing the body from absorbing about 25 percent of fat ingested. This fat is passed through the body as feces instead of being absorbed into the body. The manufacturer claims that Alli can boost weight loss by a whopping 50 percent more than diet and exercise alone. This figure is considerably

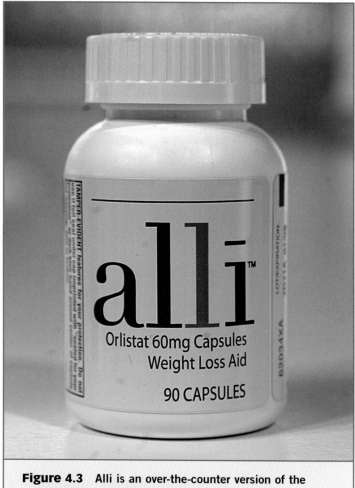

Figure 4.3   Alli is an over-the-counter version of the lipase inhibitor orlistat. (© AP Images)

higher than the 5 to 10 percent loss that most prescription drugs purport to offer.

Despite the advertised 50 percent additional weight loss, sales have been less than spectacular due to the side effects, which include loose stools, gas, oily spotting, and frequent hard-to-control trips to the bathroom. At one time, the drug's

Web site warned users that, "until you have a sense of any treatment effects, it is probably a smart idea to wear dark pants, and bring a change of clothes with you to work."[1] The manufacturers suggest that patients restrict their intake of fat to a mere 15 grams per day to reduce chances of the side effects. A typical chocolate candy bar could easily contain 15 grams of fat. One pharmacist interviewed about Alli's potential popularity quipped that he was going to put them next to the adult diapers and recommend that consumers buy one of each. Low sales would suggest that the potential for an embarrassing episode outweighs the benefit of losing a few additional pounds.

BLOCKING THE FAT: OLESTRA

Orlistat was not the first drug developed to increase weight loss by blocking fat. Olestra was created by Proctor and Gamble in 1968, originally developed as a fat substitute to increase fat intake for premature babies. This use of Olestra was a failure but Proctor and Gamble quickly realized that Olestra could have beneficial purposes for people trying to lose weight.

Olestra is made up of sugar and fat molecules that cannot be broken down by enzymes in the body. Bacteria in the intestines also will not eat it so it simply passes out of the body through the bowels. Because the body cannot absorb Olestra, its consumption prevents fat absorption. In 1996, the FDA approved Olestra for use in snack foods. As with orlistat, people who ate Olestra-containing chips, crackers, and other products experienced unsavory side effects such as abdominal cramping, severe diarrhea, and incontinence. Although the manufacturer never admitted that Olestra was linked to these side effects, word spread and sales of Olestra-containing products slumped. Consumer complaints never led the FDA to revoke its approval of the product, but Olestra has very little presence in today's snack foods.

LIMITING FAT INTAKE WITHOUT DRUGS

The easiest way to reduce fat absorption without drugs is to limit the intake of fat-laden foods. As a rule, avoiding fried foods and butter- and oil-rich sauces will reduce fat in a person's diet. The easiest way to achieve a low-fat diet without becoming obsessed with counting calories and fat grams is to shift toward a diet rich in plant-based foods such as fresh fruits and vegetables.

A diet rich in plant-based foods is also healthier. According to the American Institute for Cancer Research, a plant-rich diet is strongly associated with a cancer-protective benefit. Vegetarians, in fact, have a lower incidence of both cancer and obesity when compared with the general population. When maintaining a healthy weight, the occasional splurge is not as crucial as daily eating habits.

5

Fen-Phen and Redux: The Making and Unmaking of Drugs

In 1996, Mary Linnen was a happily engaged 29-year-old living in Massachusetts. Like many women planning a wedding, Mary decided she wanted to lose some weight, perhaps a dress size or two, to fit into her wedding dress. Her doctor prescribed a new and popular diet drug combination called Fen-phen. After just a couple weeks of taking this drug, she experienced shortness of breath and dizziness while on a golf outing with her family. Roughly a week after the outing, Mary stopped taking Fen-phen. She had been on Fen-phen a total of 23 days. Mary began to feel better, but soon her symptoms returned, and they worsened every day. She was very perplexed about what was happening to her. She felt dizzy and constantly out of breath. Seven months after she took her first Fen-phen pill, Mary went to the emergency room and had many respiratory tests done. Finally, a specialist told her she had primary pulmonary hypertension (PPH). Mary's PPH was attributed to her use of Fen-phen.

The weight-loss drug Fen-phen was pulled from the market in 1997, after it was shown to cause PPH in patients who had formerly been in good health. PPH is a rare disease where the blood vessels of the lungs get more and more narrow. Narrow blood vessels result in higher blood pressure and can lead to heart failure. It is extremely difficult to control this rare condition. Mary was promptly fitted with a chest tube and a drug to make her heart pump faster, in the hopes of delivering more oxygen to the lungs. Full recovery from PPH is nearly impossible, and patients typically survive for four years after diagnosis. Mary died a few months later, a mere 10 months after first taking Fen-phen. Mary was just one of a few people who previously had no heart conditions and developed PPH after taking Fen-phen.

FEN-PHEN

Fen-phen gets its name from a combination of two previously FDA-approved weight-loss drugs: fenfluramine and phentermine (Fen-phen). Fenfluramine was sold under the trade name Pondimin and was approved by the FDA in 1973 to suppress appetite. Like many of the first weight-loss drugs, Pondimin was meant for short-term use. These early weight-loss drugs were intended for use during a few weeks or months to jump-start a long-term weight-loss program. These weight-loss drugs did not undergo any scrutiny as long-term medication, so the FDA approved them for short-term use. Many consumers were not fond of the drowsiness that Pondimin caused. To offset this unpleasant side effect, researchers looked to combine the ingredient in Pondimin with another FDA-approved drug, phentermine.

Phentermine, which was approved by the FDA in 1959, stimulated the metabolism to burn calories. By combining these two drugs, doctors believed that patients would have their appetite suppressed and metabolism boosted without feeling sluggish. Doctors began combining these drugs as an off-label use of weight-loss medication in the 1990s. Off-label refers to a drug being used for a purpose not approved by the FDA, and therefore not listed on the drug's label. Although the FDA states a specific purpose for the drug, it is legal for physicians to use their own judgment when using a drug in a way that is not specifically listed on the label.

In August 1997, an article in *The New England Journal of Medicine* by Dr. Heidi Connelly of the Mayo Clinic revealed her experience treating women with pulmonary hypertension and heart-valve abnormalities.[1] Dr. Connelly reported 24 cases of unusual heart valve disease in patients taking Fen-phen. The patients had been taking Fen-phen anywhere from one to 28 months. Dr. Connelly felt the damage to the valves was due to the excessive amounts of serotonin that the drugs created. Other scientists echoed Dr. Connelly's concerns; eventually the findings were so obvious that a link could not be denied.

Fen-phen was eventually pulled from the market on September 15, 1997, when doctors evaluating echocardiograms from patients found that 30 percent had abnormal results. Fen-phen consumers subsequently entered into one of the largest mass lawsuits in U.S. legal history.

DRUG COMBINATIONS:
ADVANTAGES AND DISADVANTAGES

Any medication has the potential for side effects. One individual taking a medication could feel dizzy, another person might feel drowsy, and a third person might experience no side effects. In some cases, an additional drug can be added to a patient's regimen to offset the undesirable side effects, as was the goal with adding phentermine to fenfluramine to create Fen-phen. Users felt drowsy using fenfluramine alone, but no longer had this problem when they also took phentermine. Unfortunately, the combination of the drugs also created lung and heart valve damage that neither drug causes on its own.

Combining drugs without knowing the drug interactions can be highly toxic, as it was for Libby Zion. In 1984, Libby was an 18-year-old college student from New York who was taking a prescribed antidepressant, phenelzine, which increases serotonin levels. Libby went to the hospital with a fever of 103.5 and was given a narcotic painkiller Demerol to control her extreme shaking from the fever. Demerol, similar to phenelzine, also increases serotonin levels. Libby developed **serotonin toxicity** from these dangerously high levels of serotonin that caused her to become agitated. Forty-five minutes after Libby was given Demerol, the toxicity caused her to thrash about. The doctor and nurse used a restraining jacket and also tied down Libby's arms and legs to restrain her. Libby was given a sedative but her temperature soared to 108 degrees and she was dead within the next hour. A coroner's analysis also indicated that Libby may have taken cocaine earlier in the evening, which also increases serotonin levels. Libby did not tell the emergency room doctors that she had taken any other drugs; otherwise, they would not have administered Demerol.

It was debated in court what exactly killed Libby—the combination of drugs causing a toxic amount of serotonin in her body or an uncontrollable virus. Although the exact cause of her death remains unclear, Libby definitely suffered from serotonin toxicity caused by multiple drugs that increase serotonin levels. Libby's death underscores the importance of disclosing all drug use—prescription, over-the-counter, or even illegal substances—to medical professionals. Failing to divulge this information or to heed warnings on drug labels, even for over-the-counter drugs, can lead to medical complications or even death.

REDUX: TOO GOOD TO BE TRUE

In 1995, scientists gathered in a large conference room to decide whether the FDA should approve Redux (dexfenfluramine). Before the FDA will approve a drug, there are hearings where scientists and other industry experts can oppose or support a pending drug. In 1995, Dr. Leo Lutwak was the lead FDA medical officer reviewing the diet drug Redux. Lutwak thought Redux was too risky for what he thought was modest weight loss and did not think the FDA should approve it. He was concerned about the drug's effect on the brain and its "frightening" association with pulmonary hypertension.[2]

At the very least, Dr. Lutwak requested a black box on the Redux's label. The black box is a solid black border at the top of the label that would alert doctors to a potentially life-threatening risk. The manufacturer convinced the rest of the members against the black box. After hearing all of the evidence, the FDA's committee took a vote on whether to approve Redux. The committee originally voted against the drug, with five votes opposing the drug and three approving it. One member pleaded for another vote. At the next vote, members voted in favor by just one vote, with six approving the drug and five opposing it.

SEROTONIN: WHEN IS IT TOO MUCH OF A GOOD THING?

Serotonin toxicity, also known as serotonin syndrome, is a form of poisoning caused by taking too much of one drug or a combination of drugs so serotonin levels increase to life-threatening levels. Antidepressants, opiates, herbs, CNS stimulants, or any other drug that increases serotonin levels can cause this toxic state if inappropriate amounts or combinations of these drugs are taken. Serotonin toxicity can only occur from drug consumption; the central nervous system could not spontaneously release a toxic amount of serotonin without cause from a drug.

Serotonin toxicity is difficult to identify both because it mimics other medical conditions and because there is no lab test to determine if a person has this condition. Serotonin is a neurotransmitter, responsible for communicating messages in the brain. Serotonin toxicity can occur within minutes of taking an excessive amount of serotonin-boosting drugs, with symptoms including sweating, dilated pupils, tremors, twitching, muscle rigidity, and fever. Patients with serotonin toxicity often have a change in mental state, such as becoming highly agitated, feeling confused, and even hallucinating. It makes sense that disrupting the balance of this chemical would cause disruptions to normal mental and physical functions. However, it is not known why an excess of serotonin has these particular effects on the body.

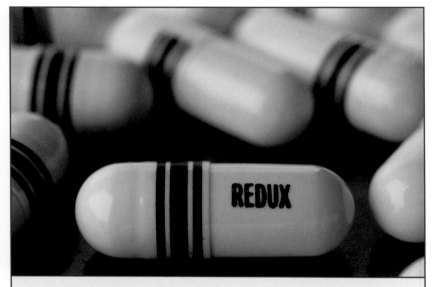

Figure 5.1 Redux was pulled from the market in 1997 because it was shown to damage the heart valves of users. (© James Leynse/CORBIS)

The FDA approved Redux on April 29, 1996. Redux's label stated that safety had not been shown for longer than one year of use. In the first full year after which Redux was approved, 18 million prescriptions were filled, with few of the prescribing doctors aware of the potential dangers. It was not until patients began reporting problems that doctors noticed a trend.

A medical technician in Fargo, North Dakota, noticed that the echocardiograms of young women taking Redux who had reported health problems looked suspicious. These women, who previously had no history of heart disease, had test results showing severely damaged heart valves. The technician became concerned and talked to the consulting doctor. The doctor also became concerned and decided to send the files to the Mayo Clinic for review. This medical technician was the first outsider to observe what would later become the very reason the FDA pulled Redux from the market in September 1997.

DEXFENFLURAMINE

Dexfenfluramine is the active ingredient in Redux. Chemically, it is very similar to the fenfluramine in Fen-phen. Redux is occasionally referred to as half of Fen-phen or "dexfen-phen." Dexfenfluramine suppressed appetite by triggering the body to release chemicals, most notably serotonin, from nerve endings that make a person feel more full.

Dexfenfluramine was often prescribed along with phentermine, similar to fenfluramine being prescribed with phentermine as Fen-phen. Combining dexfenfluramine with phentermine was an off-label use of the drug. In addition, some doctors prescribed dexfenfluramine with phentermine as a long-term weight management strategy; this was also off label because the FDA had approved these drugs only for short-term use. Dexfenfluramine was implicated in heart and lung disorders, such as primary pulmonary hypertension and heart valve disease.

What made scientists think this drug was safe? The safety of Redux was based on a one-year European study of 1,000 people; half received Redux, and the other half received a placebo or no treatment. The study population was comprised of 80 percent women with an average age of 41. According to the FDA, heart disease was not noted in the study but it was not clear what tests were administered to make sure the heart was not affected. No follow-up studies on heart disease were ever completed on these test subjects. Interestingly, dexfenfluramine had been marketed in Europe for more than a decade without a reported link with heart valve problems. This history likely influenced the approval of Redux by the FDA. In addition, doctors never suspected this drug of causing lung and heart problems; changes in heart valves, for example, are so rare that clinical trials for Redux would not have checked for this side effect. The history of Redux underscores that there are risks associated with taking even FDA-approved drugs, and that the benefits of a drug should be weighed accordingly.

DYING TO BE THIN

Despite the potentially dangerous side effects of Redux and Fen-phen, many dieters were distraught when these products were pulled from the market. Marlena Bendt, a 65-year-old woman from Illinois who struggled with weight her whole life, lost 70 pounds on Fen-phen. When she heard that the drug had been recalled, she vowed to travel to a country where it would be legal. Marlena felt she could not live without Fen-phen and definitely would not be able to keep the weight off without it.

Introducing weight-loss drugs and then revoking them can set the stage for a black market, which allows people to purchase, sell, and consume drugs that are not legal in the United States. Most of these black market purchases take place through the Internet. Procuring medication in this way is clearly dangerous to a consumer, who is unlikely to do so under a doctor's care. A prescription generally requires a trip to a doctor, at least when the medication is first prescribed. The doctor evaluates the patient to make sure that taking a certain drug will not pose any danger to the patient or conflict with any other medications that he or she is already taking.

Many of the Internet-based "pharmacies" do not require a prescription, even for legal drugs. Some Web sites assert this fact proudly, and, not unsurprisingly, there have been reports of medications that have caused a heart attack because of the prior medical condition of the individual. Other Web sites require purchasers to fill out a questionnaire and state that answers will be evaluated; often, however, there is no proof or information about the identity or qualifications of the supposed reviewer. The safety of the questionnaire method also requires that the person answers the questions truthfully; however, it would be easy for a patient who is eager to get a weight-loss drug to understand the "correct" answers. In addition to regulating the safety, effectiveness, and manufacturing of pharmaceutical drugs, the FDA also regulates the prescribing process. Specifically, the sale of a prescription drug must accompany a prescription. The FDA can prohibit Web sites that do not require a prescription from selling drugs in the United States. Because many of these companies are based outside of the United States, however, the FDA cannot shut down the sites.

6

Stimulants

Trent is a junior varsity wrestler and hopes to make the varsity team by next year. He has been training hard at the gym to prepare for a meet this weekend. If he could only lose an additional eight pounds, Trent would qualify for a lower weight class, which would make him more competitive. One of his wrestling friends recommended some pills from a health food store. The label on the bottle said the pills were natural so Trent assumed they must not be bad for him. After a few days of taking the pills, however, he started to feel nervous, he could not sleep at night, and his sister kept insisting that he was cranky.

Weight-loss drugs that act as stimulants are meant to speed up the body's metabolism. Unfortunately many of these drugs stimulate other organs that should not be stimulated, such as the heart. Stimulants such as ephedra have been implicated in more than a dozen deaths.

CAFFEINE

Caffeine is the stimulant found in coffee, tea, cola nut, maté, and guarana. Like prescription appetite suppressants, caffeine stimulates the central nervous system. Caffeine boosts energy, increases mental alertness for a limited duration, and helps to burn fat. Proponents of caffeine as a fat-burning supplement also claim that caffeine can buffer muscle pain, enabling an individual to work out longer. Too much caffeine can also have adverse health effects such as insomnia, anxiety, irritability, and in women, breast cysts.

Caffeine is often combined with other weight-loss dietary supplements, including other ephedra-like stimulating drugs such as desert tea, country mallow, Sida cordifolia, and heartleaf. For

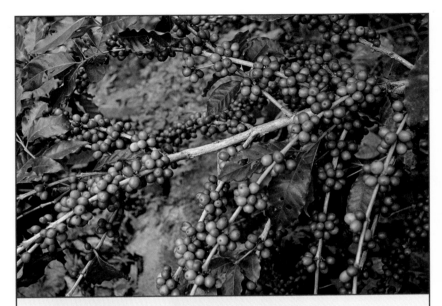

Figure 6.1 Coffee beans, shown here, contain caffeine, a stimulant. Caffeine is a common ingredient in many weight-loss supplements because it gives a slight boost in energy, although not enough to cause significant weight loss. (© Rafael Ramirez Lee/Shutterstock)

many users, it might not be clear exactly how stimulating the supplement is because ingredients such as country mallow may sound benign. Some supplements have so much caffeine that consuming one could equate to drinking as many as 32 cans of caffeinated cola in one day![1] The manufacturers of these dietary supplements also do not need clearance from the FDA to verify the safety of their products. Although caffeine might offer a temporary energy boost, it is unlikely to assist in a notable weight loss.

LAXATIVES

Dieters use laxatives as a quick way to lose weight. Some over-the-counter products that are promoted as a "dieter's tea" contain natural laxatives such as senna. Laxatives stimulate nerve endings in the **colon**, which is one of the last organs in the digestive track. Many dieters think that laxatives prevent them from absorbing a considerable number of calories from their food, but this is untrue. By the time the food has entered the colon, the body has already absorbed the majority of calories. According to Anorexia Nervosa and Related Eating Disorders, Inc., in one experiment, a group of laxative abusers ate a high-calorie meal consisting of several thousand calories. Another group ate the same meal. The laxative abusers took laxatives and the second group took nothing. Researchers collected the entire product that passed through the bowels and tested each for calorie content. The laxative abusers were only able to remove about 100 calories from their bodies, a small percentage of a meal totaling several thousand calories.[2]

Long-term abuse of laxatives is destructive to the body's natural systems and can even be fatal. Laxatives deplete the body of necessary minerals such as potassium, calcium, and sodium, as well as eliminating water. Calcium facilitates the contraction of heart muscles and potassium is necessary for the relaxation of heart muscle. Sodium is vital for maintaining fluid balance in body tissues. If these minerals are severely depleted by the purging of body fluids by laxatives, basic bodily functions such as nerve impulses, muscle contraction, and heart function can be disrupted. Prolonged use can weaken the heart, and in very rare cases even a young person could have a heart attack.

Another significant problem with laxatives is disruption of normal bowel activity. Constant stimulation of the nerve endings in the bowels from laxatives can cause them to stop responding to stimulation, even when the stimulation is natural. The laxative abuser begins to need more laxatives for the same result and eventually becomes dependent on them to have a bowel movement. Laxatives also damage the colon from the constant muscle contraction; the muscles become overstretched, resulting in constipation, gas, and possibly irritable bowel syndrome. Laxatives can also remove the protective mucus lining and therefore subject the body to a greater chance of infection. For those chronic users who decide to stop using laxatives, they will need to see a doctor to help them stop.

HERBAL FEN-PHEN

Herbal Fen-phen is a dietary supplement that contains ephedra and Saint John's Wort. Referring to this combination of drugs as herbal Fen-phen implies that the drugs will speed up the metabolism and suppress appetite just as Fen-phen did. As a dietary supplement, though, the manufacturer of this product does not need to support its claims with clinical trials.

Saint John's Wort is a supplement that is also used to treat depression. Although it is not fully understood how the compounds in this plant alleviate depression, it is believed that Saint John's Wort works by increasing levels of serotonin in the body by preventing nerve cells in the brain from reabsorbing serotonin. If the serotonin is not reabsorbed, then it is more plentiful. It is unclear how well this drug really works to alleviate depression, although it is likely most effective in mild to moderate cases. Another side effect of these increased levels of serotonin is appetite suppression. In this capacity, Saint John's Wort is meant to act like fen (fenfluramine) in the Fen-phen combination.

One proven side effect of Saint John's Wort is **photosensitivity**. Photosensitivity is a condition where a light-skinned person or animal becomes more sensitive to sun exposure and can burn more easily. Photosensitivity by users of Saint John's Wort is very rare; however, light-skinned cows eating the Saint John's Wort plant in a pasture can easily eat enough of the plant to develop photosensitivity, causing the light areas of their skin to peel off in layers while the dark areas remain unharmed. Supplements of Saint John's Wort, however, do not contain enough of the active ingredient, **hypericin**, to cause photosensitivity.

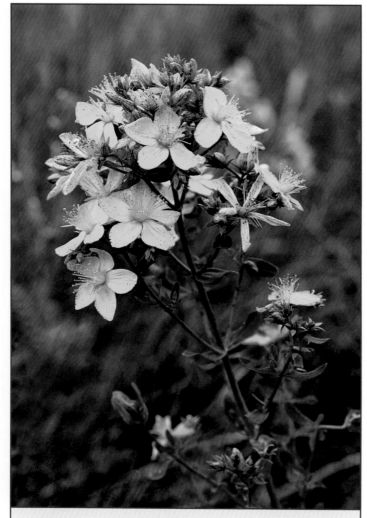

Figure 6.2 Saint John's Wort, shown here, is a plant that is one of the ingredients in herbal Fen-phen. (© Gala Khan/Shutterstock)

Ephedra is a drug that stimulates the central nervous system and burns fat while giving the user energy. Ephedra in herbal Fen-phen is meant to replace phen (phentermine) because it acts as the stimulating aspect of the drug combination. Ephedra is potentially fatal if taken in large doses or by someone with heart problems.

Herbal Fen-phen has not undergone clinical trials or any other valid scientific regimen to prove its effectiveness or safety. At best, scientific studies of the supplements indicate that Saint John's Wort does raise serotonin levels, and that ephedra stimulates the central nervous system and can, with side effects, cause a modest amount of weight loss. Studies on the combination of these drugs do not exist, and two drugs taken together can have an entirely different effect on the body than if each drug is taken alone. The FDA and Natural Products Association, the largest nonprofit group dedicated to the natural products industry, makes no claims about the safety or effectiveness of these drugs when used together.

EPHEDRA

In 2003, 23-year-old athlete and expectant father Steve Bechler was training with the hopes of becoming a pitcher for the Baltimore Orioles. In an effort to enhance his performance, he allegedly took three ephedra pills on an empty stomach. Under the heat of the sun later that day, he collapsed and died. Although Steve Bechler may have had a previously undetected medical condition such as a heart problem, ephedra is believed to have contributed to his death. Bechler is one of the many people who have died from taking too much ephedra.

Ephedra is the active ingredient in supplements such as TrimSpa, Xenadrine RFA-1, and countless other supplements available on the Internet. This controversial weight-loss drug was originally derived from the Chinese herb ma huang. The Chinese discovered the stimulating properties of this drug 2,000 years ago. The active compounds are located in the plant's stem and include ephedrine and pseudoephedrine. Ephedra has been used to treat asthma, colds, and flu, because it relaxes bronchial smooth muscles and therefore relieves shortness of breath. Ephedra is also very popular for its supposed athletic enhancement and weight-loss capabilities.

Ephedra is a natural source of ephedrine and pseudo-ephedrine, which are both CNS stimulants specifically causing the heart rate and metabolism to increase. Ephedrine and pseudoephedrine heat up the body in a process referred to as thermogenesis. During thermogenesis, the body burns more fat. Ephedrine can also increase stamina, which has made the supplement popular with body builders and other athletes. Studies show that taking ephedra on a consistent basis for a period of weeks or months results in greater weight loss than placebo. According to the National Institutes of Health, Office of Dietary Supplements, ephedra plus herbs containing caffeine was associated with a weight loss of 2.1 pounds per month for up to four months of use. Part of this weight loss could be attributed to an individual's ability to work out more or longer due to the increased stamina from ephedra.

The stimulant property of ephedra also has its disadvantages. Similar to other CNS stimulants, ephedra has been shown to cause headaches, irritability, aggressiveness, and heart palpitations, and has been associated with strokes, seizures, high blood pressure, and heart attacks. According to a review by the National Institutes of Health, ephedra is associated with higher risks of mild to moderate heart palpitations, psychiatric and upper gastrointestinal effects, and tremors and insomnia, particularly when taken in combination with a stimulant, including caffeine. Another review by the National Institutes of Health showed that people taking 32 milligrams (mg) of ephedra per day experienced a significantly higher rate of bleeding strokes than did nonusers. Some ephedra-containing dietary supplement labels recommend daily doses of up to 100 mg.[3]

Ephedra is in an unusual category in terms of regulation. When ephedra comes directly from the plant as an extract, it is classified as a dietary supplement like vitamins, minerals,

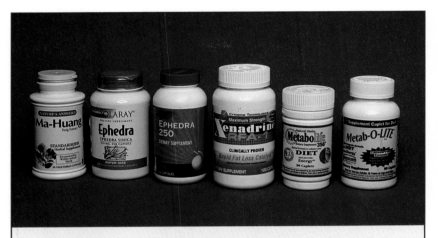

Figure 6.3 Ephedra, derived from the ma huang plant, was once found in many different over-the-counter diet aids. The FDA eventually banned the use of ephedra in dietary supplements because of its side effects. (© Leonard Lessin/Photo Researchers, Inc.)

amino acids, and other herbs. As a dietary supplement, ephedra does not have to be approved by the FDA before being sold. Only after the product reaches the market can the FDA ban the product; it is also at this point that the burden of proof of the product's safety shifts from the manufacturer to the FDA.

Ephedrine, on the other hand, is a synthetic form of ephedra, meaning that it is synthesized rather than naturally occurring in a plant; therefore it is considered a drug and is subject to FDA approval before it can be sold. Ephedrine is used in over-the-counter drugs to treat asthma, nasal congestion, and minor eye irritation. The concentration of ephedrine in these over-the-counter drugs is generally smaller than many of the ephedra supplements that were associated with health problems. It is important to remember that with any drug, dose is critical in determining the impact on health.

FDA Ban on Ephedra

Due to the mounting evidence that ephedra presented a risk to public health, the FDA took action to ban dietary supplements that contain ephedra by 2004. The ban did not include drugs that contain chemically synthesized ephedrine, traditional Chinese herbal remedies, or herbal teas containing ephedra because these products are not considered dietary supplements and are regulated differently.

The FDA ban of dietary supplements containing ephedra was the last of many steps taken by the FDA to regulate this drug based on reports of ephedra's ill effects. Prior to the ban, the FDA took action through recalls, warning letters, seizures, and criminal prosecution of manufacturers of these products. The ban of ephedra by the FDA was a first for a dietary supplement. Unfortunately, the complete ban on ephedra was not upheld in federal court nearly a year after the ban took effect.

In April 2005, a federal judge struck down the FDA ban on ephedra. A Utah supplement company, Nutraceutical International Corp., initiated the lawsuit, claiming that ephedra had been used by millions of people and was safe. The U.S. District Judge agreed with Nutraceutical International Corp. that the FDA was regulating ephedra as a drug rather than as a dietary supplement. The ruling was that the FDA cannot prevent the sale of supplements containing ephedra in doses that do not exceed 10 mg. This ruling was later reversed, banning ephedra's use in weight-loss supplements.

SYNEPHRINE

Synephrine is derived from the fruit of a plant (*Citrus aurantium*) and is chemically very similar to ephedrine. Supplements listed with bitter orange contain synephrine, which has caused a similar biological reaction, including rapid heart rate and elevated blood pressure. With the restrictions on ephedra, synephrine is being promoted without any regulations on doses. Advertisements for synephrine on the Internet claim that it has the same fat-burning, energy-boosting, and appetite-suppressing capabilities as ephedra without the "crash." Although this drug is chemically similar to ephedra, the FDA cannot ban it or regulate doses without following the same process they did for ephedra. Until then, buyers most use their own discretion.

ABUSE OF PRESCRIPTION DIET DRUGS

Prescription diet drugs are also subject to abuse and addiction. According to the International Narcotics Control Board (INCB), the drug watchdog of the United Nations, diet drugs are being abused to feed society's desire to stay slim with potentially fatal consequences. The Internet makes it much easier to abuse diet drugs.

In parts of Europe, Africa, and South Asia, prescription drug abuse has escalated to the point that people are trading these substances in larger quantities than "traditional" trafficked drugs such as cocaine and heroin. The unregulated markets in these countries make it much easier for these drugs to be brought into the United States. In President Bush's 2008 National Drug Control Strategy, he stated that while youth drug use declined by 24 percent, the illegal use of prescription drugs was becoming a growing threat. As of 2008, legislation was pending in Congress to address the problem of "rogue online pharmacies" that allow consumers to purchase prescription drugs without a prescription.

ABUSE OF DIET DRUGS IN CONNECTION
WITH AN EATING DISORDER

On the world's largest "pro-anorexia" Web site, people—mostly teenage girls—post comments bemoaning that bagel they should not have had, inquire about the best way to fast without fainting, ask how many calories 10 green grapes contain, and recommend diet drugs. Pro-anorexia Web sites support and encourage the behaviors of people with **anorexia nervosa**. Many members, of whom there are more than 16,000, admit using Adderall, a stimulant often used to treat attention deficit hyperactivity disorder (ADHD) to help them lose weight, even though their profiles of height and weight put them well into the underweight category. It is not clear if a doctor is prescribing these pills, but these pro-anorexia Web site members are clearly using them to encourage their eating disorder. The Internet also creates an opportunity for people with an eating disorder to purchase prescription weight-loss drugs, such as clenbuterol.

People with eating disorders often abuse over-the-counter weight-loss drugs. Laxatives are one of the most commonly reported drugs used, particularly stimulant-type laxatives that result in watery diarrhea. The loss of significant amounts of water, although extremely dangerous, gives the individual an immediate sense of weight loss, even though most of the calories from food are absorbed before reaching the intestines. The abuse of ephedra and ephedrine is particularly dangerous by people suffering from an eating disorder. According to research by the Mayo Clinic, ephedrine's usual recommended maximum dose is 120 mg, but the mean daily dose among five of the patients studied was 1,450 mg.[4] Two of these five patients had an eating disorder. Many sufferers use these stimulants not only as a weight-loss drug but also to provide energy during periods of fasting or very low-calorie dieting. Given the fragile health condition of many people with an eating disorder, ephedra and ephedrine taken at higher-than-recommended doses present an even greater threat than to the general population.

STIMULATING THE METABOLISM NATURALLY

The body's metabolism can change throughout the day, and drugs are not the only way to make it speed up. Exercising is the most obvious way to speed up the metabolism and increase serotonin levels without drugs. To maximize fat burning, a medium level of exercise is recommended, such as when you are working up a sweat but not having difficulty breathing. A high level of intensity, such as when you are breathless and unable to speak, is recognized by your body as an emergency situation, requiring a quick burst of energy. In this scenario, the body will use sugar from the bloodstream and also the small amount of sugar stored in muscles. Too much high-intensity exercise can cause blood sugar levels to dip too low, which causes fatigue. In addition, it is more crucial to burn fat than sugar if one is overweight. The body will access fat to burn as fuel during medium-intensity exercise.

Many treadmills, elliptical machines, and stationary bikes offer a rough idea of how many calories a person is burning based on the age and weight of the person and provide a heart rate monitor to help the person gauge the intensity of the workout. Twenty minutes of an elliptical machine workout will be a bigger boost to a person's metabolism than any drug available.

What these machines do not calculate, however, is the boost in metabolism after stepping off the machine and moving on with the day. Even while a person is cooling down, the metabolism is still revved up. In addition, the most profound benefit a workout gives to the metabolism is the increase in muscle mass from working out. By adding muscle mass, the body will have a higher basal metabolism. Whereas taking many stimulants is likely to cause side effects that make a person feel miserable, working out is a beneficial alternative that will make him or her feel fabulous.

7

Going Off Label for Weight Loss

An "off-label" use of a drug occurs when it is prescribed to treat a condition that is not specifically listed on the label. The U.S. Food and Drug Administration (FDA) is the agency that mandates what disease a drug can be marketed to treat, and this information is printed on the label; however, it is legal for physicians to use their own judgment when prescribing drugs off label.

FDA AND DRUG APPROVAL

The FDA determines whether a drug should be approved, and for what purpose. Drugs must undergo a considerable amount of research before they can be considered for approval. Drugs undergo clinical trials by being tested on people. When the manufacturers of a drug believe they have enough evidence to show that their drug can treat a condition without a significant threat to human health, they present their research to the FDA's committee of medical specialists; these researchers investigate whether to approve or reject a drug.

When the FDA gives approval to a drug, it also determines the conditions that the drug can claim to treat. A drug that gets approval from the FDA for reducing blood pressure cannot be marketed for another purpose unless the drug makers get approval for this additional condition. Getting approval to market a drug for an additional condition or disease requires years of research. In the interim, doctors can use their own judgment when prescribing a drug in a way that is not specifically listed on the label without fear of breaking the law. Some physicians have been criticized, however, for prescribing some drugs, such as those intended to treat ADHD, to treat weight loss.

THE ORIGINS OF OFF-LABEL USES

Often a drug is found to treat a condition merely by accident. For example, Rogaine, which is a hair-loss treatment, was originally used to treat high blood pressure. While performing experiments on people, researchers noticed that patients were growing hair on their shoulders, legs, head, and other areas of the body. The researchers then decided to apply some of the product on their arms to see if hair growth increased. After several months, there was a noticeable increase in hair growth. Many years later the makers of Rogaine were able to receive permission from the FDA to market the drug as a prescription treatment for hair loss. The use of Rogaine to promote hair growth prior to its approval by the FDA would be considered an off-label use. Prescribing a drug for an off-label use is legal but in some situations can raise ethical concerns.

Many drug makers do not seek FDA approval to get additional uses added to their drug's label. The reason is essentially financial. Getting FDA approval can require millions of dollars spent on research to prove safety and effectiveness for the new use. If a drug manufacturer believes that the off-label use is well known by doctors, then there is little incentive to seek FDA approval in order to expand the marketing of the drug. Another reason that off-label use might perpetuate without FDA approval for the additional use is if the target market is relatively small. A cholesterol-lowering drug has a large potential market because so many people struggle with cholesterol. If this cholesterol drug was suddenly found to treat a less widespread condition, such as boils, there would be little incentive for a drug maker to spend money to get this new use approved to target individuals who might seek drug treatment for their boils.

The disadvantage to off-label use is that that FDA has not granted approval, which leaves consumers at a slightly greater risk. Fen-phen is a good example of the dangers of off-label uses of drugs. Although fenfluramine (fen) and phentermine (phen) were both previously approved by the FDA, combining these drugs was an off-label use. Another off-label use was combining phentermine with dexfenfluramine (Redux). In addition, the FDA had approved fenfluramine and phentermine for short-term use, but doctors were allowing patients to stay on these medications indefinitely. The combination of these drugs and the duration of use contributed to the heart valve disorders that caused these drugs to be deemed unsafe and pulled from the market.

Another significant disadvantage of taking medications off label is that an insurance company might not cover the drug for that purpose. Arlene Bartolett, who lives in Pennsylvania with a severely diseased liver and only one-third of her liver function remaining, is very familiar with this dilemma. A liver transplant might be in her future, but for now she relies on a drug called CellCept. CellCept's label use is as an antirejection drug meant for organ transplant patients. Doctors discovered that CellCept also helped keep a diseased liver functioning, and this became an off-label use for CellCept. In 2006, Bartolett's health insurance provider notified her that they would no longer pay for her off-label use of this drug. CellCept costs approximately $800 for a 90-day supply. Bartolett appealed this decision and she was issued provisional coverage of the medication while the insurance company reviewed the case. In the interim, Bartolett cut her dosage in half to spread out what she had. She began to feel tired and her doctors became concerned. Bartolett won her appeal and was approved for another year of coverage for CellCept through her prescription plan. After receiving media attention in 2008, Bartolett's insurance provider changed their approval from one year to "indefinitely." Although Bartolett won her battle to get coverage for an off-label use of a drug, it is likely that other people are less fortunate.[1]

OFF-LABEL DRUGS FOR WEIGHT LOSS

Adderall is an amphetamine that can increase blood pressure and heart rate and is used to treat ADHD. Similar to other amphetamines, such as prescription appetite suppressants, Adderall has the side effect of suppressing appetite, resulting in weight loss. Adderall's label states that the drug treats ADHD. The off-label use is weight loss, which is why it was prescribed for Alex Veith.

Veith was 11 years old and 30 pounds overweight. Veith's blood test showed that he was likely to develop type 2 diabetes if he continued on the same path of weight gain. His parents claimed that he was active and eating a healthy diet and therefore felt their only other option was to seek medical attention.

Veith was prescribed Adderall and lost weight, eventually maintaining a normal weight. Veith was thrilled with his weight loss and claimed he felt full all the time. Veith's parents were also happy with the results of Adderall. Veith took Adderall for four years, consistently maintaining a healthy weight and never developed diabetes. At 18 years of age, Veith had stopped taking Adderall but had not gained weight.[2]

Dr. John Lantos, professor of pediatrics at the University of Chicago, believes that prescribing ADHD medications off label for weight loss is medically and morally questionable. The debate is whether it is acceptable to prescribe a drug not approved for weight loss when the drug may have serious side effects. The FDA warns that patients with heart problems have suffered sudden death when using ADHD drugs. Due to these concerns, in April 2008, the American Heart Association recommended that children should be screened for heart problems with an **electrocardiogram** (EKG) before being prescribed drugs to treat ADHD. If the EKG detects an abnormal rhythm of the heart, then the stimulant would not be prescribed to the child. The FDA also links Adderall with psychiatric problems such as hearing voices and manic behavior. The doctor who prescribed Adderall for Veith, Dr. Ziai, screens his patients for heart problems and indicates that psychiatric side effects occur in only 2 percent of his patients. For this 2 percent, Dr. Ziai

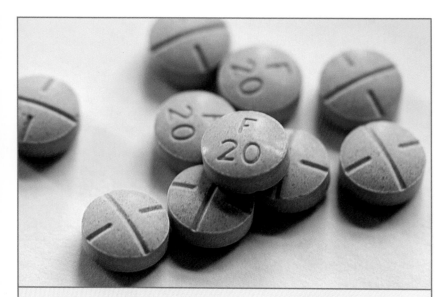

Figure 7.1 Adderall's original use is to treat ADHD, but it has begun to be used off label as a weight-loss drug. (© Chris Gallagher/Photo Researchers, Inc.)

lowers the dose and then raises it once the child's body has had a chance to adjust.[3]

Scientifically backed statistics on how much weight loss Adderall, or any other ADHD drug, is likely to cause are not available. Research does not have to be submitted to the FDA for an off-label use, so doctors can often rely only on anecdotal evidence rather than data to judge whether the drug works. Dr. Ziai, who only treats children and teens, has prescribed Adderall for about 800 children and teens and has seen weight loss in 90 percent of them. Dr. Ziai's observation of his patients is an example of anecdotal evidence, whereas a clinical trial would be scientific data. Doctors such as Ziai support the use of Adderall for obese children in cases where there are no other medical solutions to the child's weight problem. These doctors believe in the benefits of preventing type 2 diabetes, as well as other obesity-related illnesses.

ANTIDEPRESSANTS

Like many prescription appetite suppressants, many antide-pressants treat depression by increasing levels of serotonin in the body. The discovery of antidepressants that encourage weight loss is a victory for people who suffered weight gain while on their medications to treat depression. In fact, weight gain was a significant disadvantage to many of the previously available mood-stabilizing medications.

With many antidepressants, patients commonly experience an initial weight loss followed by a steady gain. It is difficult for doctors to determine to what extent the weight loss or gain results from the depression subsiding. If a person begins to feel less depressed, he or she may eat more (or less) depending on how he or she responds to depression. In some cases, antide-pressants might just reestablish a patient's normal eating habits. Some scientists feel that antidepressants play a greater role in weight gain or loss than just the effect of relieving depression. One theory is that antidepressants that cause weight gain might make the body more resistant to insulin and leptin. As for anti-depressants that cause weight loss, the increase in serotonin is believed to suppress appetite. Similar to other weight-loss drugs, though, the body can adapt to the drug and any weight loss ben-efit can cease. Bupropion and sertraline are the two antidepres-sants most associated with weight loss.

Bupropion

Bupropion was FDA approved in 1988 but a newer, extended-release formulation was created in 2003 by GlaxoSmithKline under the trade name Wellbutrin XL. Sales of Wellbutrin have been impressive, totaling $1.4 billion in 2005. Bupropion is prescribed off label for weight loss.

After repeatedly observing that depressed patients lost weight, scientists decided to test bupropion's weight-loss capabilities on people who were overweight but were not depressed. In a study by Duke University that was paid for by the makers of Wellbutrin, approximately two-thirds of the participants lost 5 percent of their body weight within the first eight weeks. Those patients who continued to take the bupropion for another 16 weeks lost an average of 12.5 percent of their body weight, a similar percentage of weight loss attributable to drugs labeled for weight loss.

Prescribing bupropion off label for weight loss has its critics. The main criticism is that the long-term safety and effectiveness of going off label for weight loss has not been determined. Doctors who prescribe bupropion for weight loss tell their patients that they'll probably need to take the drug for life. Some medical professionals support off-label use of drugs to control obesity because minimizing the risk of obesity-related diseases outweighs the potential dangers of long-term use and the side effects of a drug. Bupropion's side effects include abdominal pain and anxiety.

Sertraline

Sertraline, a popular antidepressant manufactured by Pfizer under the trade name Zoloft, increases serotonin levels in the body. The FDA approved Zoloft in 1991. In clinical trials, patients were found to have a very short-term weight loss due to a decreased appetite. This short-term weight loss is typically two to three pounds in the first six weeks. Over the long term, though, sertraline can make patients gain weight for reasons that are not well understood.

Interestingly, sertraline has been found to be particularly helpful for obese patients who suffer from **night eating syndrome**. People with night eating syndrome overeat in the evenings, eat little or nothing in the mornings, and awake throughout the night to eat, consciously yet with a difficult-to-resist urge. In an eight-week study of 34 patients with this syndrome, the mean weight loss in overweight and obese subjects was 6.4 pounds.[4]

SEIZURE MEDICATIONS

Theresa Saleeby was 31 when she told her doctor that she wanted to lose 50 pounds. Her doctor prescribed the seizure medication Topiramate as an off-label weight-loss aid. In the next seven months, she said she suffered from memory loss, her legs falling asleep, and her hair falling out in golf ball–sized clumps. In addition, she only lost 3 pounds.

Topiramate is made by Ortho-McNeil and sold under the trade name Topamax. Topamax was approved by the FDA in 1996 to treat seizures. The current label shows that it is approved for the treatment of seizures and as a daily medication to prevent migraines. Topiramate has the side effect of weight loss and is therefore also being prescribed as a weight-loss drug as an off-label use. Topiramate users, even those not struggling with weight, report a significant decrease in appetite.

For seizures, topiramate helps to calm the brain cells that are working much more rapidly than they should during a seizure. It is not entirely clear why topiramate works to control migraines and to suppress the appetite, but the management of seizures, migraines, and appetite takes place in the brain, which is why this drug is used for all three conditions.

Topiramate is not considered a good choice for weight-loss treatment due to the side effects, such as memory loss and difficulty concentrating. Many users report feeling sluggish while taking topiramate, although this side effect is likely to improve as the body adjusts to the medication. Other serious side effects include kidney stones due to topiramate's tendency to increase the acidity of the blood. For those with seizures or severe migraines, the potential side effects are likely worth the benefits. As a weight-loss drug, however, these side effects raise concerns and will likely limit topiramate from being advertised as a weight-loss drug.

All drugs have side effects and potential risks. Taking drugs off label may pose additional risks because the FDA has not approved the off-label use. Doctors must use their discretion when prescribing off-label uses for their patients, but ultimately the patient must decide if the modest weight loss justifies the side effects.

8

The Future of Weight-Loss Drugs

Marcy was one of those women perpetually on a diet. She had tried everything including high-protein diets, low-fat diets, and lemon and tomato juice diets, but she still had those residual 15 pounds to lose. Then Marcy heard about a hypnosis seminar as a drug-free alternative for weight loss. The cost of the seminar was $59.99 but the ad claimed that participants could lose 120 pounds a year. And Marcy only needed to lose 15 pounds! The ad also claimed that she would experience "34 high-powered, fat-eliminating suggestions best described as a deliberate and systematic bombardment of fat destroying technology."

Once Marcy attended the seminar, however, the focus quickly turned from hypnosis to supplements such as TrimSpa. The sponsors of the seminar were New Jersey–based Goen Technologies, manufacturers of TrimSpa, LipoSpa, and CarbSpa. Marcy was told that TrimSpa would remove the extra glucose and blood sugar that her body produces when she overeats or eats fattening foods and direct it to her muscles where it would be used as energy instead of being stored as fat. This claim is simply false. Marcy and the other seminar participants were urged to make purchases of a single bottle for $44.95 or the fabulous deal of $459.99 for a 16-pack supply of supplements with a 110 percent money-back guarantee if they were not satisfied. Fortunately for Marcy, she did not fall for these gimmicks and left the seminar, having wasted only $59.99.

WEIGHT-LOSS CLAIMS: FACT VERSUS FICTION

Marcy is just one of many dieters who have paid money believing outrageous claims about weight loss. In Marcy's situation, there was some vindication. In 2003, the founder of Goen Technologies was later sued by the New Jersey Office of the Attorney General for false claims through tactics including these seminars. The complaint filed by the State of New Jersey lists the false claims made by Goen Technologies. No scientific evidence exists that TrimSpa metabolizes appetite or regulates blood sugar. Goen also claimed that CarbSpa "reduces absorption of carbohydrates" and that LipoSpa "sucks the fat right out of food you eat before it can get to your hips, thighs, waist, neck, or arms." In addition to these wildly false claims, the complaint also alleged that consumers did not get the 110 percent money-back refund they were promised. Perhaps the most serious allegation was that the makers of these products used ephedra without disclosing its dangers, thereby putting their consumers at a health risk. Unfortunately, these types of scams are not uncommon. Buyers should follow the advice that if a weight-loss product sounds too good to be true, it probably is.

CLINICAL TRIALS

Clinical trials play a pivotal role in the final stages of drug research. A clinical trial is a research study using humans, not animals, to answer health questions, usually in an attempt to get a new drug or use approved by the FDA. Clinical trials are completed in four phases, with each phase meant to answer a research question and advance the drug closer to approval. Phase I of a clinical trial involves testing the drug on a small group of people for the first time to evaluate its safety, determine appropriate dosage, and identify any side effects. Phase II is a similar process with a larger test group of 20 to 300 people. Phase III involves administering the drug to a large group of 300 to 3,000 people to evaluate effectiveness, compare it to

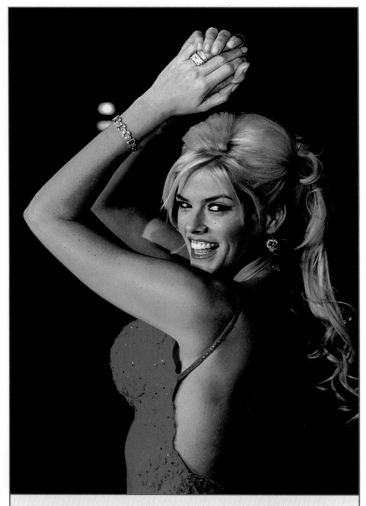

Figure 8.1 Anna Nicole Smith was a spokesperson for TrimSpa, which she claimed helped her to lose more than 50 pounds. No scientific evidence backs up TrimSpa's weight-loss claims. (© AP Images)

commonly used treatments, examine side effects, and collect additional data to ensure that the drug is safe and effective. Generally, completion of two successful Phase III trials is required for FDA drug approval. Phase IV clinical trials take place after the drug has been marketed; researchers conduct studies to evaluate both the drug's effect on different populations and any potential long-term side effects. If harmful effects are discovered in this phase, then the drug may become restricted to certain uses or may no longer be sold. One case of Phase IV trials resulting in an FDA recall was Vioxx, a previously FDA-approved drug used to treat arthritis that was found to produce harmful side effects, specifically risks of heart attack and stroke.

The researchers are responsible for informing the participants in a study about potential risks. The ultimate decision is left to the patient. So why might someone be willing to be a human guinea pig? Money is one possibility. Patients are often paid for participating in a trial. Another patient might wish to receive a treatment without paying for it, which might be the case with a weight-loss drug. A third scenario might be a participant with a disease that has not responded to other drugs who is willing to try something new through the clinical trial. For example, an AIDS patient might try many drugs to treat his or her disease. If someone suffering from AIDS is not responding to approved medications and an experimental drug becomes available, that person might be inclined to enter a clinical trial in the hopes that this new drug might alleviate his or her condition.

AN INVERSE MARIJUANA: RIMONABANT AND TARANABANT

Rimonabant and Taranabant are closely related drugs that control appetite with a mechanism similar to, or perhaps opposite of, the way marijuana stimulates hunger or the "munchies." Neither of these drugs is approved for use in the United States, but Rimonabant is a popular drug in Europe, made by a French company named Sanofi-Aventis and sold under the trade name Acomplia. Unfortunately, both Rimonabant and Taranabant can be unlike marijuana in another way, causing depression, rather than the euphoria associated with cannabis.

Rimonabant

Rimonabant works by blocking a **receptor** in the brain that influences the regulation of body weight, glucose, and lipid metabolism. By blocking this receptor, Rimonabant is believed

SLIM CHANCE AWARDS

Each year, the Weight Loss Abuse Task Force reviews the many weight-loss gimmicks and highlights the most fraudulent ones. The "award" is meant to highlight the prevalence of false claims in the weight-loss industry. The 2006 award for Worst Product went to PediaLean, which is a fiber capsule meant for overweight children. The product was advertised in tabloids and magazines, including *Redbook* and the *National Enquirer*. The active ingredient is glucomannan, which is a soluble fiber that can absorb up to 200 times its weight in water, thereby making a person feel more full. The problem with glucomannan is that it swells in the body, which causes cramping and discomfort and can also create an obstructive mass in the intestines. The ads promoted PediaLean as safe, but it is one of the weight-loss products for which the Federal Trade Commission is requiring a settlement for deceptive claims.

The 2006 Most Outrageous Claim was awarded to Isacleanse. The ads for Isacleanse promoted a product as a detox. Detox refers to detoxification, specifically of unhealthy chemicals that proponents claim accumulate in the body and cause a variety of ailments, including weight gain. The idea that any over-the-counter supplement can "detox" the body is fraudulent. The body is naturally self cleaning. Isacleanse ads offered pills and teas with the promise of a leaner body in 30 days. There is nothing new about trying to lose weight and maintain that weight loss, and no new drug can guarantee long-term weight loss.

to reduce the craving to eat more. If the brain is not receiving the signal to eat, then a person simply will not have as strong an impulse to eat. Clinical trials have shown that one-third of patients lose 10 percent of their body weight, similar to the results with sibutramine and orlistat. Studies from the University of Alberta in Canada have also shown that Rimonabant can also reduce blood pressure and cholesterol levels.

Scientists developed this drug based on their knowledge of drugs that stimulate certain areas of the brain lead to an increase in appetite. One example of these appetite-stimulating drugs is marijuana. Research into these areas of the brain, known as the cannabinoid receptors, led them to understand that this same area of the brain could also control other cravings like nicotine. Unfortunately, controlling the areas of the brain that also regulate pleasure, pain, and relaxation had a downside that prevented the drug from getting FDA approval.

A scary potential side effect is an increased risk of mood disorders such as depression and anxiety. Researchers from the University of Alberta found a 6 percent increased risk of psychiatric problems while on this drug. Another study published in the November 2006 medical journal *Lancet* looked at 4,000 patients who were taking either Rimonabant or a placebo. Patients were not told whether they were receiving the real thing so they would not be biased. In addition to the patients not knowing what they were receiving, the doctors giving the pills were not told by the experimenters if the pills they were administering were the real drug or the imposter. This is another way to prevent bias in an experiment and is referred to as a **double blind experiment** because neither the patient nor the person administering the medication knows who is getting the drug.

In this study, patients receiving Rimonabant were 2.5 times more likely than their sugar pill–consuming counterparts to discontinue the study due to depressive disorders. They were also three times as likely to stop taking the drug because of anxiety.[1] Four patients committed suicide while taking Rimonabant: Three were taking the drug during clinical trials and one person was a European taking the drug after it was approved. The concern over these disorders led the FDA advisory board to rule unanimously (14–0) not to recommend Rimonabant for approval to the FDA in 2007. The biggest fears of panel members were the increased risk of suicidal tendencies from taking this drug. Sanofi-Aventis issued a statement after the decision, indicating that they would continue to work with the FDA advisory panel to address concerns about the drug. Although Rimonabant is not legal in the United States it was approved by the European Drug Agency in June 2006, which means it is legal in Europe.

Taranabant

On a pharmaceutical blog, people, mostly scientists, post comments about the likelihood of Taranabant getting FDA approval given the history of Rimonabant. On an April 8, 2008, posting, Jennifer writes, "I was briefly on the clinical trial for this drug. I don't know what dosage I received, however, I was compelled to stop the drug after three weeks because of 'nervous system effects.'" Jennifer further writes that she flew into fits of rage for mundane occurrences such as being given incorrect change at the grocery store. Her husband found her shaking and crying on the floor in the closet; she became suddenly disoriented and unable to distinguish home from work. And then there were the thoughts of suicide. Jennifer writes that she never experienced anything like this before, and that her symptoms abated as soon as she stopped taking the drugs. Although she lost 12 pounds in 3 weeks, she gained all of it back.[2]

Jennifer's experience reflects the concern many doctors have about drugs that tamper with the **endocannabinoid system** of the brain, specifically the increase in psychiatric symptoms including suicidal tendencies. The endocannabinoid system controls appetite, pain, pleasure, and mood. Taranabant is made by Merck and is currently navigating clinical trials in the hopes of an approval by the FDA advisory board. Merck is aiming for a 5 percent weight loss to satisfy the FDA with its effectiveness. The drug is able to yield the 5 percent weight loss but only at its highest dosage of 4 mg, which also caused side effects similar to Rimonabant. By lowering the drug's dosage to 2 mg, these side effects lessened but the drug lost its effectiveness.

Many scientists express doubt that the FDA will ever approve Taranabant because it is chemically very similar to Rimonabant, and therefore likely to produce psychiatric side effects. Based on comments on a pharmaceutical blog, some scientists question why a well-regarded company such as Merck would try to get approval for Taranabant despite its serious side effects. The lucrative billion-dollar weight-loss market will, no doubt, continue to motivate drug companies to discover new weight-loss drugs—that do not produce serious side effects.

LORCASERIN

Lorcaserin is promoted by its manufacturer, Arena Pharmaceuticals, as having all the benefits of Fen-phen without any of the potential damage to heart valves. As of 2008, lorcaserin is nearing the end of its Phase III clinical trials without any damage to the heart by its users. Lorcaserin is the chemical name with the brand name to be determined.

Similar to Fen-phen, lorcaserin stimulates the production of serotonin causing users to feel full. Fen-phen caused heart valve damage by stimulating a specific receptor (the 2B receptor) that causes fibrous deposits to form on the heart valves. Lorcaserin, instead, stimulates the 2C receptor at 100 times more than the 2B receptor.[3]

People taking lorcaserin lost eight pounds during a 12-week period. Participants in the experiment had significant testing of their hearts and were found to suffer no adverse effects. If lorcaserin gets approved by the FDA, Arena is likely to enjoy a billion dollar profit; if the drug is not approved, lorcaserin will be another example of the FDA refusing to take a chance on a weight-loss drug.

DRUGS, THE INTERNET, AND THE FDA

Many people today feel comfortable making purchases over the Internet, even of prescription drugs. The Internet serves as a pharmacy that can ship products globally. With new Internet drug companies popping up almost daily, the FDA warns about the possible dangers of purchasing prescription drugs in this manner.

In 2007, the FDA received complaints that a counterfeit weight-loss drug was sold to three consumers on two different Web sites. The sites claimed to be selling Xenical, an FDA-approved drug meant for obese patients who meet specific height and weight requirements. Lab tests eventually showed that the product sold did not contain any of the active ingredients found in authentic Xenical. Instead, the pills contained the active ingredient sibutramine, which is contained in Meridia, another weight-loss drug. It is impossible to discern whether the pills were inadvertently or intentionally switched. Whatever the case, such a switch can be extremely dangerous to a patient.

The FDA also discovered that other samples from these Web sites contained only talc and starch, despite the valid lot number that appeared on the packaging. A lot number indicates specifics of where the drug was manufactured, but the lot number listed on the drug did not correlate with the true expiration date for that lot. The expiration was listed as April 2007, whereas the expiration date of the lot was March 2005. Further investigation revealed that these two Web sites had been implicated previously in selling counterfeit drugs to fight avian bird flu. Both of these companies are based outside the United States. The FDA recommends that consumers exercise caution when buying any drugs over the Internet, especially if there is no way to contact anyone at the Web site by phone or if the drugs seem much cheaper than usual.

The National Association of Boards of Pharmacy (NABP), which was created in the early 1900s to help states develop

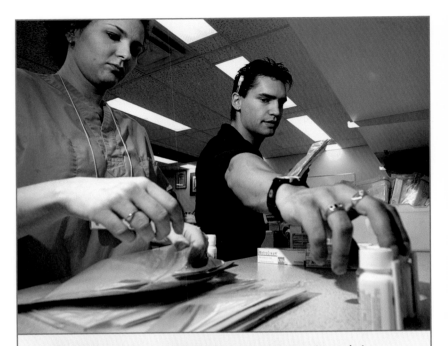

Figure 8.2 Internet pharmacies have sprung up to market weight-loss drugs and other prescription medications to consumers. Many of these companies are unscrupulous, selling fake drugs or filling falsified prescriptions. Only online pharmacies that are certified Verified Internet Pharmacy Practice Sites (VIPPS) should be considered for medication purchases over the Internet. (© AP Images)

medical licensing standards, responded to irresponsible Internet pharmacies by creating a certification program to prove which Web sites are legitimate. This certification program requires that an Internet site selling prescription drugs maintain all state licenses, honor patient privacy, and allow the NABP to inspect its operations. By following these requirements, the Web site can then provide documentation of the certificate—Verified Internet Pharmacy Practice Sites (VIPPS)—so customers know that the site has been reviewed and approved by a group of independent doctors.

WEIGHING THE OPTIONS—AND RISKS

Weight-loss drugs are a popular choice among many dieters. The weight-loss product market in the United States alone is estimated to reach $61 billion in 2008.[4] Weight-loss drugs, however, rarely provide a permanent solution to excess pounds. Although most of these drugs are meant for short-term use and only result in minimal weight loss (not exceeding 5 percent), many people are willing to encounter the side effects. In the case of ephedra and Fen-phen, these side effects were severe or fatal for some users. The FDA does not approve over-the-counter weight-loss supplements, so users must either self-monitor their health or seek a physician's assistance. Even after the FDA banned ephedra, lower doses of ephedra and chemically similar supplements such as synephrine have been widely available.

Weight-loss drugs are in significant demand despite the Fen-phen and Redux debacles. With nearly one-third of Americans obese and two-thirds overweight, weight-loss drugs have a large audience; this population drives pharmaceutical companies to spend billions of dollars to develop a drug with the effectiveness and popularity of Fen-phen without the damaging side effects. The disadvantage of taking almost any weight-loss drug is that the body adapts, which leads the person to experience a weight-loss plateau. Weight-loss drugs might offer an incentive to the significantly overweight, but only a permanent lifestyle change of diet and exercise will benefit one's health in the long run.

Notes

CHAPTER 1

1. Mary L. Gavin, M.D., "Overweight and Obesity," *KidsHealth*, http://www.kidshealth.org/parent/general/body/overweight_obesity.html, accessed April 8, 2008.
2. CDC, "About BMI for Adults," http://www.cdc.gov/nccdphp/dnpa/healthyweight/assessing/bmi/adult_BMI/about_adult_BMI.htm, accessed November 7, 2008.

CHAPTER 2

1. Malcolm Ritter, "Fat Belly and 40? Your dementia risk is rising," *Bucks County Courier Times* (March 27, 2008): 1A, 7A.
2. "Little bit of fat not so bad: new study," theage.com.au, November 8, 2007, http://www.theage.com.au/articles/2007/11/08/1194329391171.html, accessed January 12, 2008.
3. Steven Reinberg, "Genes May Spur Some Childhood Obesity," MedicineNet.com, January 17, 2007, http://www.medicinenet.com/script/main, accessed February 12, 2008.
4. Colette Bouchez, M.D., "The Dream Diet: Losing Weight While You Sleep," WebMD, Reviewed January 1, 2007, http://www.webmd.com/sleep-disorders/guide/lose-weight-while-sleeping, accessed March 23, 2008.

CHAPTER 3

1. Steven R. Peiken, M.D., *The Complete Book of Diet Drugs* (New York: Kensington, 2000), 75.
2. Ibid., 77.
3. Peiken, "Meridia FAQ," Obesity-news.com, http://www.obesity-news.com/merfaq.htm, accessed March 2, 2008.
4. Ginger Thompson, "Bushman Squeeze Money From a Humble Cactus," *The New York Times*, April 1, 2003, http://www.williams.edu/AnthSoc/native/san.htm, accessed February 2, 2008.
5. Ginger Thompson, "Hoodia," Drugs.com, http://www.drugs.com/hoodia.html, accessed February 2, 2008.

6. Ginger Thompson, "Kiera Knightley BMI is way too low," *Star Diet Secrets* online, http://stardietsecrets.com/keira-knightley-bmi-is-way-too-low, accessed April 6, 2008.
7. Ginger Thompson, "Clenbuterol for Weight Loss Hits Hollywood," *Fit and Healthy* online, http://ifitandhealthy.com/clenbuterol-for-weight-loss, accessed March 30, 2008.
8. Katy Guest, "Clenbuterol: The new weight-loss wonder drug gripping Planet Zero," *The Independent*, http://www.independent.co.uk/life-style/health-and-wellbeing/health-news/clenbuterol-the-new-weightloss-wonder-drug-gripping-planet-zero-441059.html, accessed April 2, 2008.
9. Rebecca Howard, "The size zero pill," *The Daily Mail*, October 9, 2005.
10. Salynn Boyles, "Drinking Water May Speed Weight Loss," WebMD, January 5, 2004, http://www.webmd.com/diet/news/20040105/drinking-water-may-speed-weight-loss, accessed December 8, 2007.

CHAPTER 4

1. Danny Adler, "Limited Demand for New Diet Pill," *Bucks County Courier Times* (June 17, 2007): 1C–5C.

CHAPTER 5

1. Kate Cohen, "Fen Phen Nation," PBS's *Frontline*, Web edition, November 13, 2003, http://www.pbs.org/wgbh/pages/frontline/shows/prescription/hazard/fenphen.html, accessed October 30, 2007.
2. Susan Kelleher, "Rush toward new weight-loss drugs tramples patients' health," *The Seattle Times*, July 14, 2005.

CHAPTER 6

1. Dr. Rob, "Energy Boosters are not natural," *Bucks County Courier Times* (April 22, 2008): 2D.
2. Anorexia Nervosa and Related Eating Disorders, Inc., "Laxatives and enemas: not the way to go," March 24, 2007,

Notes

http://www.anred.com/lax.html, accessed March 2, 2008.

3. Carol Rados, "Ephedra Ban: No Shortage of Reasons," *FDA Consumer magazine*, March–April 2004, http://www.fda.gov/FDAC/features/2004/204_ephedra.html, accessed April 24, 2008.

4. J.A. Tinsley and D. D. Watkins, "Over-the-counter stimulants: abuse and addiction," *Mayo Clinic Proceedings* 73 (1998): 977–982.

CHAPTER 7

1. Guy Petroziello, "Against doctor's orders: Rx for disaster," *Bucks County Courier Times* (March 4, 2008): 6A.

2. Elizabeth Cohen, "ADHD drug use for youth obesity raises ethical questions," CNN.com, http://edition.cnn.com/2007/HEALTH/03/21/vs.adderall/index.html, accessed March 29, 2008.

3. Ibid.

4. Laurie Barclay, M.D., "Sertraline May Be Effective for Night Eating Syndrome," Medscape.com, May 11, 2006, http://www.medscape.com/viewarticle/532147, accessed May 8, 2008.

CHAPTER 8

1. Gupta Sanjay, M.D., "Diet-Pill Dilemma," *Time* 170, 24 (December 10, 2007): 76.

2. Derek Lowe, "Taranabant in Trouble?" *In the Pipeline*, March 12, 2008, http://pipeline.corante.com/archives/2008/03/12/taranabant_in_trouble.php, accessed May 13, 2008.

3. Alexis Madrigal, "New Weight-Loss Drug Like Fen-Phen, But Not As Heart Breaking," *Wired Science*, January 9, 2008, http://blog.wired.com/wiredscience/2008/01/weight-loss-dru.html, accessed May 1, 2008.

4. Madrigal, "Obesity Treatment Gives You the Opposite of the Munchies," *Wired Science*, January 8, 2008, http://www.wired.com/print/medtech/drugs/news/2008/01/reverse_cannabis, accessed May 1, 2008.

Glossary

amphetamines—A group of drugs that stimulate the central nervous system, causing mental or physical functions to speed up.

anorexia nervosa—An eating disorder characterized by extremely low consumption of food and resulting in low body weight.

catecholamines—A group of neurotransmitters that signal a flight-or-fight response in the body.

central nervous system—The brain, nerves, and spinal cord.

central nervous system stimulants—Drugs that can speed up mental or physical functions.

chronic—A medical condition that is continuous.

colon—The largest organ in the digestive system that is stimulated by laxatives.

diabetic neuropathy—Nerve damage due to diabetes that causes tingling or loss of feeling in the body.

dietary supplement—A pill, capsule, powder, or liquid that supplies nutrients such as vitamins or minerals.

double blind experiment—A scientific experiment where neither the patient nor the person giving the drug knows which pills represent the drug being tested or the placebo.

electrocardiogram—A test that records the electrical activity of the heart to detect any abnormal rhythms.

endocannabinoid system—An area of the brain that controls appetite, pain, pleasure, and mood.

flight-or-fight—A biological response to stress characterized by the release of stress hormones that cause a variety of changes in the body such as appetite suppression.

gene defect—A general term for a gene that causes the body to operate in an undesirable way, generally leading to disease.

ghrelin—A hormone produced in the gastrointestinal tract that stimulates appetite.

high-fructose corn syrup (HFCS)—A sweetener manufactured from corn syrup that is a common additive in processed foods.

hypericin—The active ingredient in Saint John's Wort.

hypothalamus—An area of the brain that controls a number of bodily functions, including appetite.

insulin—A hormone produced by the pancreas that takes sugar from the bloodstream and enables the body to use it as energy.

Glossary

ketosis—A state where the body burns stored fat instead of carbohydrates.

leptin—A hormone that binds to the hypothalamus and signals the body to feel full.

lipase—An enzyme that breaks down fat.

metabolism—The body's process of creating and using energy to support functions such as breathing and digesting.

neurons—Cells in the brain and spinal cord that transmit information.

neurotransmitters—Chemicals in the brain that act as messengers between neurons.

night eating syndrome—An eating disorder where a person overeats in the evenings, eats little or nothing in the mornings, and awakes throughout the night to eat.

off-label—A drug being used for a purpose not approved by the FDA.

osteoarthritis—Pain in the joints as a result of abnormal wearing of the cartilage.

photosensitivity—A condition of heightened sun-sensitivity in light-skinned people and animals.

placebo—A pill containing an inert substance such as sugar. Placebos are used in experiments to evaluate the change in a person's condition based on his or her expectation of receiving treatment.

plateau effect—The leveling off of weight loss while a consistent regimen of diet and exercise that previously produced weight loss is being maintained.

processed foods—Food such as white bread, where the plant fiber, and most of the nutrition, has been removed from the grain.

receptor—A protein on the cell that binds to a molecule, such as a neurotransmitter.

serotonin—A neurotransmitter that promotes a feeling of well-being.

serotonin toxicity—A form of drug poisoning from medications that raise serotonin levels to levels that can cause fever, rapid heart rate, muscle spasms, and even death.

trade name—A name for a specific product brand.

weight-loss drug—Any over-the-counter or prescription drug used for weight loss.

Bibliography

Barr, Naomi. "Maybe You Need to Gain 10 Pounds." *O, The Oprah Magazine*, February 2008, 108.

Campos, Paul F. "Dying to be thin: Killed by a culture bent on beauty." *Bucks County Courier Times*, February 28, 2008, 9A.

Canelli, Rachel. "Enjoying the fruits—and veggies—of their labor." *Bucks County Courier Times*, January 16, 2008, 1B–3B.

Dzubow, Lauren. "Sour News on Sweetener." *O, The Oprah Magazine*, February 2008, 108.

Hellmich, Nanci. "One-third of U.S. kids are out of shape, study finds." *USA Today*, October 3, 2006. Available online. URL: http://usatoday.com/news/health/2006-10-02-us-kids-unfit_x.htm. Accessed May 12, 2008.

Henkel, John. "Buying Drugs Online: It's Convenient and Private, but Beware of 'Rogue Sites.'" *FDA Consumer*. Available online. URL: http://www.fda.gov/fdac/features/2000/100_online.html. Accessed August 5, 2007.

Koepke, Tracey. "Long-Term Study Finds Antidepressant Effective for Weight Loss in Women." *DukeMed News*, September 11, 2001. Available online. URL: http://www.dukemednews.org/news/article.php?id=3652. Accessed September 15, 2007.

Law, Bridget Murray. "What's Ahead for Rimonabant?" *Doc News*, September 1, 2007. Available online. URL: http://docnews.diabetesjournals.org/cgi/content/full/4/9/10. Accessed May 13, 2008.

Liu, Simin. "Whole-grain foods, dietary fiber, and type 2 diabetes: searching for a kernel of truth." *American Journal of Clinical Nutrition* 77 (2003): 527–529.

Marcovitz, Hal. *Diet Drugs*. Farmington Hills, MI: Thomson Gale, 2007.

Neporent, Liz. "Diet Pills and Teens." AOL Diet and Fitness. Available online. URL: http://body.aol.com/diet/basics/diet-pills-teens. Accessed February 12, 2008.

Saul, Stephanie. "F.D.A. Panel Rejects Drug for Obesity." *The New York Times*, June 14, 2007. Available online. URL: http://query.nytimes.com/gst/fullpage.html?res=9C0CE7D9143FF937A25755C0A9619C8B63&partner=rssnyt&emc=rss. Accessed May 13, 2008.

Further Resources

Books

Barrett, Cece. *The Dangers of Diet Drugs and Other Weight-Loss Products*. New York: Rosen, 1998.

Kausman, Rich. *If Not Dieting Then What?* Melbourne, Australia: Allen and Unwin, 2005.

Marcovitz, Hal. *Diet Drugs*. Farmington Hills, MI: Thomson Gale, 2007.

Ojeda, Linda, PhD. *Safe Dieting for Teens*. Alameda, CA: Hunter House, 2007.

Walker, Pamela. *Understanding the Risk of Diet Drugs: A Teen Eating Disorder Prevention Book*. New York: Rosen, 2000.

Web Sites

Centers for Disease Control and Prevention BMI Calculator
http://apps.nccd.cdc.gov/dnpabmi/Calculator.aspx

Drug Digest
http://www.drugdigest.org

eMedicineHealth
http://www.emedicinehealth.com

Mayo Clinic
http://www.mayoclinic.com

Quackwatch
http://www.quackwatch.org

Science Daily
http://www.sciencedaily.com

USDA—MyPyramid.gov
http://www.mypyramid.gov

U.S. Food and Drug Administration Center for Drug Evaluation and Research
http://www.fda.gov/cder/index.html

U.S. National Library of Medicine—National Institutes of Health
http://www.nlm.nih.gov

WebMD
http://www.webmd.com

Index

Index

Index

About the Author

Suellen May is a writer living in Bucks County, Pennsylvania. She received a B.S. from the University of Vermont and a M.S. from Colorado State University. She writes science-related books and magazine articles. She is the author of *Botox and Other Cosmetic Drugs* and a five-book environmental series entitled *Invasive Species*.

About the Consulting Editor

David J. Triggle, Ph.D., is a University Professor and a Distinguished Professor in the School of Pharmacy and Pharmaceutical Sciences at the State University of New York at Buffalo. He studied in the United Kingdom and earned his B.Sc. degree in chemistry from the University of Southampton and a Ph.D. in chemistry at the University of Hull. Following postdoctoral work at the University of Ottawa in Canada and the University of London in the United Kingdom, he assumed a position at the School of Pharmacy at Buffalo. He served as chairman of the department of biochemical pharmacology from 1971 to 1985, and as dean of the School of Pharmacy from 1985 to 1995. From 1995 to 2001, he served as the dean of the graduate school, and as the university provost from 2000 to 2001. He is the author of several books dealing with the chemical pharmacology of the autonomic nervous system and drug-receptor interactions, has published some 400 scientific articles, and has delivered more than 1,000 lectures worldwide on his research.